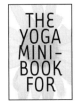

THE
YOGA
MINI-
BOOK
FOR

Stress
Relief

A Specialized Program for a Calmer, Relaxed You

ELAINE GAVALAS

Illustrations by Nelle Davis

A Fireside Book · Published by Simon & Schuster · New York London Toronto Sydney Singapore

FIRESIDE
Rockefeller Center
1230 Avenue of the Americas
New York, NY 10020

Copyright © 2003 by Elaine Gavalas

Illustrations copyright © 2003 by Nelle Davis

For information regarding special discounts for bulk purchases, please contact
Simon & Schuster Special Sales at 1-800-456-6798 or business@simonandschuster.com

Designed by Chris Welch

Manufactured in the United States of America

3   5   7   9   10   8   6   4   2

Library of Congress Cataloging-in-Publication Data
Gavalas, Elaine.
The yoga minibook for stress relief : a specialized program for a calmer,
relaxed you / Elaine Gavalas.
p.   cm.
"A Fireside book."
Includes index.
1. Stress management.   2. Stress (Physiology)   3. Yoga.   4. Relaxation.
I. Title: Yoga minibook for stress relief.   II. Title: Stress relief.   III. Title.
RA785 .G38   2003
155.9'042—dc21   2002029428

ISBN 0-7432-2701-8

This publication contains the opinions and ideas of its author. It is intended to provide helpful and informative material on the subjects addressed in the publication. It is sold with the understanding that the author and publisher are not engaged in rendering medical, health, or any other kind of professional services in the book. The reader should consult his or her medical, health, or other competent professional before adopting any of the suggestions in this book or drawing inferences from it.

The author and publisher specifically disclaim all responsiblity for any liability, loss, or risk, personal or otherwise, which is incurred as a consequence, directly or indirectly, of the use and application of any of the contents of this book.

Respectfully dedicated to
the great heroes of September 11

Acknowledgments

This book would not have been possible without the help and creative contributions of my husband and writing guru, Stuart Katz. His brilliant literary judgment and patient work helped me bring this text to life. I am forever grateful for his extraordinary love, friendship, and support.

I wish to offer my heartfelt thanks to all of the talented professionals at Simon & Schuster Trade Paperbacks for producing my yoga books series, with special thanks to Trish Todd, for providing me with the opportunity to write the books; to my editor, Lisa Considine, for her expertise and sage guidance; and to Anne Bartholomew, for her valuable assistance.

I also wish to extend my deepest gratitude and appreciation to my literary agent, Michael Psaltis (and the Ethan Ellenberg Literary Agency), for his wise counsel, encouragement, and support of my yoga books from the beginning.

I especially wish to thank Nelle Davis, who brought the yoga poses alive with her wonderful illustrations.

I am truly grateful to my parents-in-law, Ethel Katz Regolini and Leo Regolini, and my uncles, Arthur Vozeolas and Henry Kane, for their wisdom, help, and guidance.

Finally, many thanks to my yoga teachers (with special gratitude to Ram Dass), and to you, dear reader. May yoga bring you lasting health, happiness, peace, longevity, freedom, and bliss. *Om shanthi* with love.

Contents

chapter 1

Understanding Yoga

Would you like to feel more relaxed and enjoy peace of mind? Global upheaval, along with the pressures of two-career families, longer work hours, the shifting employment landscape, financial concerns, and death, illness, and divorce, has led to a worldwide stress epidemic. What can you do about your own stress?

You hold the answers to that question in your hands. I've written *The Yoga Minibook for Stress Relief* for everyone who suffers from stress-related problems such as anxiety, depression, tension, insomnia, and high blood pressure. The yoga program described in this book addresses stress relief in a unique way that merges and integrates your body, mind, and spirit. By following this program you can relieve your stress and prevent it from accumulating. You can also promote relaxation with tension-relieving yoga poses, breathing, and meditation, all while you develop a fit and beautiful physique. Yoga for Stress Relief is a lifestyle program that will help you counter stress naturally and safely, and restore balance in your body and life.

Exercise fads continue to come and go, but after more than five thousand years, the practice of yoga is still with us—and more popular than ever. Although there are many kinds of exercise programs, only Yoga for Stress Relief offers a holistic anxiety-busting combination of yoga stretching exercises *(asanas)*, deep breathing exercises *(pranayamas)*, and meditation techniques. The practice of yoga offers a positive change in lifestyle, in which stress relief, emotional wellness, and cardiovascular fitness are natural by-products of enjoyable exercise.

After taking the necessary precautions and familiarizing yourself with the basic yoga movements in Chapter 2, you'll kick off with my stress-relief program in Chapter 3. It begins with the Three Yoga Steps to Relaxation, which involve recognizing the stress, releasing the tension, and breathing deeply. Practicing yoga relaxation, breathing, and meditation shuts down the fight-or-flight stress response and triggers the parasympathetic nervous system's relaxation response. Chapter 3 explains in detail how to practice the first and second steps, recognizing stress and releasing tension. It also provides an introduction to the third step, breathing deeply with yoga breathing exercises. You'll expand practice of the final step with the meditation and mantra exercises in Chapter 4.

The Yoga Movement Meditation Workouts in Chapter 5 incorporate the three yoga steps of relaxation with *vinyasa* (a continuous flow of yoga poses) and meditation practice. This powerfully effective combination of yoga and meditation makes the most of your workout time and is a superlative way to alleviate stress and improve your cardiovascular fitness, flexibility, and strength.

Don't despair if time is short. You can rest, relax, and revitalize in just minutes with the Restorative Yoga Workout in Chapter 6. Practicing these gentle, nurturing, and healing yoga poses will soothe your body, mind, and spirit. Restorative yoga is a stress-relief workout that's good for you physically, emotionally, and spiritually. You'll also find valuable ways to unwind and relax with the soothing scents of ayurvedic aromatherapy before, during, and after your yoga practice.

The rigors of coping in today's world can overload our nervous systems. Signs of overload—including heightened anxiety, depression, irritability, fatigue, and insomnia—are all too common. The healing asanas in Chapter 7 will help you beat the blues, and they'll alleviate anxiety and bring sweet dreams.

I've found that combining yoga with self-massage can be a powerful way to help restore the body's natural balance, increase well-being, and relieve stress and tension. Throughout this book you'll find self-massage techniques, such as *do-in* and self-acupressure, incorporated into yoga postures. They're a dynamic healing duo.

Do-in and self-acupressure are Asian self-massage healing techniques that have been practiced for thousands of years. They both employ touching, tapping, rubbing, stretching, and applying pressure to move the vital life force, called ch'i (or, in the yoga tradition, prana). These techniques clear energy blockages, increase circulation, and harmonize the body. Self-massage—specifically pressing and stretching the acupressure points along meridian pathways through which ch'i flows—balances this vital energy.

For many reasons, such as illness, aging, and trauma, tension accumulates around the acupressure points, thereby obstructing ch'i from flowing properly through the body. Integrating self-massage into yoga poses helps to release this tension so that ch'i circulates freely. This not only relieves tension and prevents it from building up, but it stimulates self-healing and promotes radiant health.

Over the years, I've studied and practiced many hatha yoga styles, such as Integral, Iyengar, ashtanga vinyasa, kundalini, mantra, raja, and tantra, and have been especially interested in yoga's therapeutic applications. I've observed individuals and groups practicing yoga, and I've seen its power help people relieve stress and lose weight while they increase their energy, strength, and longevity. I've had an opportunity to apply yoga techniques to help people achieve their wellness goals, and I've observed spectacular results. I've written my yoga book series—the first four being *The Yoga Minibook for Stress Relief, The Yoga Minibook for Weight Loss, The Yoga Minibook for Longevity*, and *The Yoga Minibook for Energy and Strength*—as self-help guides in response to people's many wellness, fitness, and diet problems, questions, and concerns.

My greatest wish is to share with you the many wonderful benefits yoga practice has given to me and the individuals I've assisted over the years. Whether you're looking to relieve stress, lose weight, boost your energy, or find the fountain of youth, I've created a yoga book for you. But before we dive in, a little background.

21st-Century Yoga

Throughout the centuries, yoga has redefined and re-created itself to meet the needs of different eras and cultures. Yoga was barely known in the Western world until the 1960s, when the Beatles went off to India to find spiritual enlightenment with Maharishi Mahesh Yogi. Since then, yoga has evolved from a practice for hippie spiritual seekers chanting *om* with Swami Satchidananda at Woodstock in 1969 to a practice embraced by everyone from Hollywood stars striving for beautiful bodies and high-powered CEOs seeking stress relief, to baby boomers in search of ways to turn back the hands of time. Even United States Supreme Court Justice Sandra Day O'Connor takes a weekly yoga class. At least fifteen million Americans include some form of yoga in their fitness regimen.

Although yoga has been celebrated as the new fitness philosophy for the twenty-first century, the practice of yoga actually goes back thousands of years. Yoga originated in India and is an ancient philosophical discipline, not a religion. The original purpose of practicing yoga was to experience spiritual enlightenment, a state of pure bliss and oneness with the universe. *Yoga* is a Sanskrit word meaning "union"; it describes the integration of body, mind, and spirit, and communion with a universal energy, the Supreme Consciousness. The practice of hatha yoga, whose exercises are familiar to many Westerners, was originally devised to strengthen the body and prepare it for the long, motionless hours of meditation.

Yoga dates back to the ancient Vedas, sacred Hindu scriptures first recorded around 2500 B.C.E. Over millennia, the yoga tradition has evolved into eight principal branches, different paths that all lead to the same goal: enlightenment.

The eight branches of yoga are called the Wheel of Yoga. They include:

Hatha Yoga (pronounced *haht-ha*), the yoga of physical discipline and bodily mastery. This is the branch of yoga most of us in the West are familiar with, and it is the one presented in this book. In hatha, enlightenment is achieved through spiritualized physical practices including asanas (postures), pranayama (controlled breathing), and meditation. The *Hatha Yoga Pradipika*, a fourteenth-century text, is a guide to hatha yoga.

Jhana Yoga (pronounced *gyah-nah*), the yoga of wisdom and knowledge. In jhana, enlightenment and self-realization are achieved through the teaching of nondualism, the elimination of illusion, and direct knowledge of the divine.

Bhakti Yoga (pronounced *bhuk-tee*), the path to achieve union with the divine through love and acts of devotion.

Karma Yoga (pronounced *kahr-mah*), the path of enlightenment through selfless service and actions.

Mantra Yoga (pronounced *mahn-trah*), the yoga of sacred sounds for self-awakening. A form of mantra yoga familiar to Westerners is Transcendental Meditation (TM).

Kundalini Yoga (pronounced *koon-da-leenee*), the activation of the latent spiritual energy stored in the body and raised along the spine to the head through the breath and movement.

Tantra Yoga (pronounced *tahn-trah*), union with all that you are, achieved by harnessing sexual energy. Although tantra yoga has become famous for some rituals that spiritualize sexuality, it is essentially a spiritual discipline of nonsexual rituals and visualizations that activate spiritual energy.

Raja Yoga (pronounced *rah-jah*)—also known as royal, classical, eight-limbed, or *ashtanga* (not to be confused with the separate ashtanga style of yoga)—yoga of the mind and mental mastery. In the second century B.C.E., the great Hindu sage Patanjali

wrote down the principles of classical yoga in the *Yoga Sutras.*
Patanjali describes eight steps or "limbs" known as the Tree of
Yoga. These eight limbs provide ethical guidelines for living
and help along the yoga path to enlightenment.

The Tree of Yoga is composed of:

Yama (pronounced *yah-mah*), the roots of the tree, which are
moral discipline and ethical restraints. These include nonvio-
lence *(ahimsa),* truthfulness, freedom from avarice, chastity,
and noncovetousness.

Niyama (pronounced *nee-yah-mah*), the trunk of the tree. It is
made up of self-restraints and observances, including cleanli-
ness, contentment, self-discipline, introspection or self-study,
and devotion.

Asana (pronounced *ah-sah-nah*), the branches of the tree. It includes the postures of hatha yoga.

Pranayama (pronounced *prah-nah-yah-mah*), the leaves of the tree.
It includes breath control for circulation of *prana,* or life-force
energy.

Pratyahara (pronounced *prah-tyah-hah-rah*), the bark of the tree.
It includes withdrawal of the senses for meditation.

Dharana (pronounced *dah-rah-nah*), the sap. It includes concentration for meditation.

Dhyana (pronounced *dee-yah-nah*), the flower. It includes the practice of meditation.

Samadhi (pronounced *sah-mah-dhee*), the fruit. It is the state of pure consciousness, or total bliss. All of the limbs of yoga lead to samadhi.

Your Yoga Practice

Whether you're nine or ninety, you can enjoy and greatly benefit from practicing the yoga stress-relief program that follows. Its requirements are minimal. You need only 30 to 60 minutes each day; a nonskid mat; comfortable, nonrestrictive clothing, and a small exercise space. Turn off your phone, put on the answering machine, and let your family and friends know that you're not to be disturbed during your yoga time—unless, of course, they want to join you. You can even slip 10-minute yoga breaks into your daily schedule.

You'll notice that the practice workouts in this book include poses that stretch the spine in six directions. In yoga there is a saying, "You're as young as your spine." If you stretch your spine in six directions during your daily practice you will be richly rewarded with a youthful, flexible, strong back and body. The six directions (and some representative poses) are:

- Forward (Standing Forward Bend)
- Backward (Standing Backbend)
- Right side (Gate Pose Right)
- Left side (Gate Pose Left)
- Right twist (Crocodile Twist Right)
- Left twist (Crocodile Twist Left)

As I mentioned earlier, yoga is a noncompetitive practice. There's no need to compete with other yogis or yoginis. Simply do the best that you can each and every time you practice. Your body will respond differently to the poses done from day to day because of various factors, such as your diet, the amount of sleep you've had, and the time of day you're practicing. It is important to remember that the practice of yoga is a journey and an exploration into the nature of your self.

Practicing yoga is well worth it. If you're interested in a lifetime of calm, balance, inner peace, strength, and radiantly good health, then this is the book for you. *Namaste!* (*Namaste* is a traditional yoga blessing that means "The divine in me bows to the divine in you.")

Your Yoga for Stress Relief Program

The Yoga for Stress Relief Program includes six steps to help you prevent and relieve stress, promote relaxation, combat anxiety and depression, and get in shape in the shortest time possible. Begin with Step 1 and continue with Steps 2 through 6, according to your physical condition and capabilities. An overview of each step and practice plan follows. You can find a more detailed description of each practice plan in Chapters 2 through 7.

Step 1: Yoga Basics Practice Plan

Step 2: Yoga Relaxation and Breathing Practice Plan

Step 3: Yoga Meditation Practice Plan

Step 4: Yoga Movement Meditation Workout Plans (Beginner, Intermediate, and Maintenance)

Step 5: Restorative Yoga Workout Plans (Restorative Yoga Workout, and Maintenance Movement Meditation and Restorative Yoga Workout)

Step 6: Wellness Yoga Workout Plans (Wellness Yoga Workout, and Maintenance Movement Meditation and Wellness Yoga Workout)

STEP 1. YOGA BASICS PRACTICE PLAN

Begin with the Yoga Basics poses found in Chapter 2 and practice for 1 week. Do these poses for 20 to 30 minutes, 3 or 4 days a week. Be aware that it may take you more than 1 week to do this routine comfortably, depending on your physical condition. If you feel comfortable and confident doing these poses, proceed to Step 2, the Yoga Relaxation and Breathing Practice. Otherwise, stay with Week 1 until you feel strong enough to continue. See Chapter 2 for the detailed workout.

STEP 2. YOGA RELAXATION AND BREATHING PRACTICE PLAN

After practicing the Yoga Basics for 1 week, begin the Yoga Relaxation and Breathing Practice. This 4-week plan includes the Three Yoga Steps to Relaxation (Yoga Observation, 7-Step Yoga Relaxation Sequence, and Yoga Breathing). Practice for 30 to 40 minutes, 3 or 4 days a week. Be aware that it may take you more than 4 weeks to do this routine comfortably, depending on your physical condition. See Chapter 3 for the detailed workout.

STEP 3. YOGA MEDITATION PRACTICE PLAN

After practicing the Yoga Relaxation and Breathing routines, begin the Yoga Meditation Practice. This 4-week plan includes the Three Steps to Yoga Relaxation (Yoga Observation, 7-Step Yoga Relaxation Sequence, and Yoga Breathing), along with meditation and mantra. Practice for 30 to 40 minutes, 4 or 5 days a week. Be aware that it may take you more than 4 weeks to do this routine comfortably, depending on your physical condition. See Chapter 4 for the detailed workout.

STEP 4. YOGA MOVEMENT MEDITATION WORKOUT PLANS

After practicing Yoga Meditation, you'll begin the Yoga Movement Meditation Workout. These routines will help you relieve stress and get in shape in the shortest time possible. Each practice session includes Yoga Observation, Warm Up with 7-Step Yoga Relaxation Sequence, Sun Salutation, and Cool Down with Yoga Breathing, Meditation, and/or Relaxation poses. A walking meditation is optional. As you progress from Beginner to Maintenance over a period of 2 months and beyond, you'll build your yoga practice up from

30 to 60 minutes a day, 3 to 5 days a week. See Chapter 5 for the detailed workouts.

1. Beginner Movement Meditation Workout
Weeks 1 through 4

Start with the Beginner Movement Meditation Workout, combining Sun Salutation with ujjayi breathing for 30 to 40 minutes, 3 or 4 days a week.

2. Intermediate Movement Meditation Workout
Weeks 1 through 4

After completing the Beginner Movement Meditation Workout, continue with the Intermediate Movement Meditation Workout, combining Sun Salutation with ujjayi breathing and mantra or mindful awareness for 50 minutes, 4 or 5 days a week.

3. Maintenance Movement Meditation Workout
Week 1 and Beyond

After completing the Intermediate Movement Meditation Workout, continue with the Maintenance Movement Meditation Workout, combining Sun Salutation with ujjayi breathing and mantra or mindful awareness for 60 minutes, 5 days a week.

STEP 5. RESTORATIVE YOGA WORKOUT PLANS

The 4-week Restorative Yoga Workout can be practiced alone or in combination with the Yoga Movement Meditation Workouts. Do these poses for 10 minutes, 3 days a week. Be aware that it may take you more than 4 weeks to do this routine comfortably, depending on your physical condition. See Chapter 6 for the detailed workout.

STEP 6. WELLNESS YOGA WORKOUT PLANS

This 4-week yoga routine to help relieve depression, anxiety, and insomnia can be practiced alone or combined with the Yoga Movement Meditation Workouts. Do these poses for 10 to 20 minutes, 3 days a week. Be aware that it may take you more than 4 weeks to do this routine comfortably, depending on your physical condition. See Chapter 7 for the detailed workout.

chapter 2

Before You Begin

Before you begin your Yoga for Stress Relief Program, make a realistic assessment of your current level of health and fitness. Some of the cautions outlined below may apply to you. On the basis of your initial assessment, set some feasible stress-relief goals. Only then should you begin the Yoga Basics Practice that follows.

A Word of Caution

Yoga should never cause you pain. Due to the intense stretching involved, you need to be tuned in to your body. You should be aware of where your "edge" is in each posture—the point beyond which your body can't comfortably go any further. Your edge is *not* the point at which you feel burning pain. As you explore each yoga pose, go slowly and cautiously, finding the point to which you can stretch safely. As you gradually become stronger and more flexible, you'll find that your edge will change. You'll be able to comfortably and safely stretch further and hold the poses longer.

Before beginning any new exercise program, you should consult with your health care practitioner, especially if you have health problems or physical limitations. Also, women should be aware that practicing inverted postures, such as Half Shoulderstand and Legs-up-the-Wall Pose, is not recommended during the first few days of menstruation. If you are pregnant, be sure to obtain clearance from your physician before beginning a hatha yoga program. There are many excellent prenatal yoga classes with certified instructors that teach specific prenatal yoga routines.

Never practice yoga poses that cause you pain or discomfort. If pain persists, be sure to consult with your health care professional.

Your Stress-Relief Goals

Before beginning this yoga program, try to be clear about your stress-relief goals. How much time are you giving yourself to reach them? Set reasonable goals and know that anything worth striving for takes time. Starting with your first yoga lesson, you'll get immediate relief from stress and enjoy a relaxed mind and body. However, it usually takes a minimum of 2 to 3 months of consistent yoga practice to build up healthful habits and mental, emotional, and physical resources, all of which will help prevent future stress.

It also takes a minimum of 2 to 3 months of consistent yoga exercise before changes in strength, flexibility, and body composition (less fat and more muscle) begin to appear. Depending on your physical condition when you begin this program, it may even take 6 months or more before your body really starts to show results. You may want to begin a yoga journal and jot down your thoughts about how you look and feel to help you pinpoint areas you would like to change.

It's a good idea to check your progress every 3 months and reassess your goals. For example, after 3 months you may be finishing the Movement Meditation and Restorative Yoga Workout (in Chapter 6). At that point, you will want to determine what types of physical or emotional stress you are still experiencing. You may then decide to combine the Wellness Yoga routine with the Movement Meditation and Restorative Yoga Workout, practice Wellness Yoga alone, practice 10-Minute Restorative Yoga alone, or stay with the Movement Meditation and Restorative Yoga Workout for a while longer.

Please keep in mind that this yoga stress-relief plan is not only a workout, it's a lifestyle modification program that will build healthful habits to prevent and alleviate stress, and will improve and protect the quality of your health and appearance. Make a daily affirmation to yourself to reach your stress-relief goals through consistent yoga exercise and breathing and meditation practice.

Yoga Basics

An understanding of certain fundamental movements will help you to perform the yoga postures in this book correctly. The following basic yoga preparations are incorporated into many yoga postures and will help you build strength, flexibility, and proper alignment in your upper body and lower back.

The squeeze, hold, and release actions found in Shoulder Press and Squeeze and Pelvic Tilt are fundamental to yoga practice. They massage tension and stress out of a particular area while bringing fresh, oxygenated blood into the muscles and tissues. The lifting-the-sternum action found in Mountain Pose is repeated over and over again within many yoga postures.

The use of your core strength—the lifting of your abdominals for maximum support—is also essential while performing yoga postures. In yoga, this includes the *mula bandha*, or "root lock," which contracts the perineum, and the *uddiyana bandha*, which contracts the abdomen. The mula bandha and uddiyana bandha actions are incorporated into many yoga poses. They draw awareness to the core of your body and strengthen the core abdominal, pelvic, and genital muscles.

Ujjayi breathing is a classic *pranayama* (yoga breathing) technique. It can be combined with Sun Salutation (see Chapter 5) to link the postures together and promote concentration, calm, and meditation. Yoga Observation is the first step to Yoga Relaxation and should be included in your yoga session whenever possible to calm the mind and nervous system.

Yoga Basics Practice Plan

Begin your first week of yoga practice with the following Yoga Basics poses. Be aware that it may take you more than 1 week to do this routine comfortably, depending on your physical condition. If you feel comfortable and confident doing these poses, proceed to the Yoga Relaxation and Breathing Practice in Chapter 3. Otherwise, stay with Week 1 until you feel strong enough to continue.

Week 1

Practice Schedule: Practice Yoga Basics poses for 20 to 30 minutes, 3 or 4 days a week.

Yoga Basics Poses:

Shoulder Press and Squeeze

Mountain Pose and Lifting the Sternum

Pelvic Tilt and Modified Relaxation Pose

Chest Expander

Ujjayi Pranayama

Mula Bandha

Stomach Lift

Yoga Observation

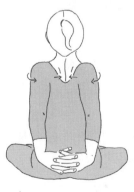

Yoga Basics Poses

SHOULDER PRESS AND SQUEEZE

What It Does: These shoulder movements are incorporated into many yoga postures, including Cobra Pose, Downward-Facing Dog, and Camel Pose. The squeeze, hold, and release actions are fundamental to yoga practice, massaging tension and stress away and bringing fresh, oxygenated blood into the muscles and tissues.

How to Do It:

1. Sit up straight on the mat with your legs crossed, arms at your sides.

2. Inhale and raise your shoulders up toward your ears. Squeeze and hold for 4 counts. Exhale and release, pressing your shoulders down and away from your ears.

3. Clasp your hands behind your back. Inhale and straighten your elbows. Press your shoulders down and away from your ears. Exhale and gently squeeze your shoulder blades together. Hold for 3 counts. Release your hands.

4. Repeat.

MOUNTAIN POSE AND LIFTING THE STERNUM (TADASANA)

What It Does: The subtle but important action of lifting the sternum, or breastbone, toward the ceiling is incorporated into many yoga postures, including Standing Backbend and Modified Head-to-Knee Pose.

How to Do It:

1. Stand tall with feet together, legs straight, and hands in prayer position over your heart center. Visualize a string attached to your sternum, or breastbone (the bone in the center of your chest).

2. Inhale and visualize the string being pulled up toward the ceiling. Feel the subtle lifting and expanding of your chest, rib cage, and sternum, lengthening the front of your body. Keep your shoulders relaxed and down, away from your ears.

3. Exhale and release.

4. Repeat.

PELVIC TILT AND MODIFIED RELAXATION POSE
(MODIFIED SAVASANA)

What It Does: These pelvic movements are incorporated into many yoga postures, including Standing Backbend, Bow Pose, Camel Pose, and Cobra Pose. The lower-back press, hold, and release actions are fundamental movements in yoga, massaging tension and stress away while bringing fresh, oxygenated blood into the muscles and tissues. Be sure to tighten the buttock muscles firmly to protect and stabilize your lower back and activate the abdominals.

How to Do It:

1. Lie on your back, knees bent and feet flat on the mat, hip-width apart. Rest your hands on your abdomen. Inhale and allow your lower back to arch naturally.

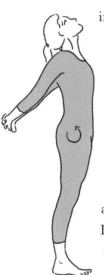

2. Exhale, tightening your buttock muscles, tilting your pelvis under, and pulling your abdomen in. Press the small of your back gently to the mat. Inhale and release.

3. Repeat.

CHEST EXPANDER

What It Does: This exercise joins together the preceding three movements: the Shoulder Press and Squeeze, Pelvic Tilt, and Mountain Pose and Lifting the Sternum. If your shoulders and chest are tight, try clasping a towel or belt behind you while doing this exercise.

How to Do It:

1. Stand with your feet hip-width apart and clasp your hands behind your back.

2. Inhale, lifting your sternum toward the ceiling as you press your shoulders down and away from your ears. Exhale, straightening your elbows and gently squeezing your shoulder blades together. Tighten the buttock muscles, tilt the pelvis under, and pull the abdomen in.

3. Inhale, release, and relax.

UJJAYI PRANAYAMA

What It Does: Ujjayi breathing is a classic yoga breathing technique. It is combined with Sun Salutation to help link the postures together and promote concentration, calm, and meditation.

How to Do It:

1. Keeping your mouth closed, constrict the back of your throat, or glottis (the opening between the vocal chords), during inhalation and exhalation. This produces a hissing sound, like that heard at the approach of Darth Vader.

2. If this is too difficult, try to whisper the sound *aaah* while in-

haling and exhaling through your open mouth. Then close your lips and breathe through your nose, continuing to make the hissing or *aaah* sound at the back of your throat.

MULA BANDHA

What It Does: The *mula bandha,* or "root lock," contracts the perineum, or pelvic floor, which comprises the pubococcygeus muscles between the rectum and genitals. This draws your awareness to the core of your body and helps build strong abdominal, pelvic, and genital muscles.

How to Do It:

1. Sit straight and tall on a chair or cross-legged on the floor. To visualize where your pelvic muscles are, imagine stopping the flow of your urine. Inhale, then exhale and contract these muscles, pulling up through your genital area and drawing up through your spine. Inhale and release the muscles.

2. Isolate the muscle group around your anus. Inhale, then exhale, contracting these muscles and drawing them upward. Inhale and release the muscles.

3. Now combine the two actions. Inhale, then exhale and con-

tract the muscles of your anus and genitals at the same time. Inhale
and release the muscles.

STOMACH LIFT *(UDDIYANA BANDHA)*

What It Does: It strengthens the abdominal muscles and keeps them
flexible, and it tones and massages the abdominal organs and glands.
Practice it on an empty stomach.

How to Do It:

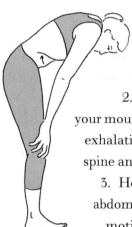

1. Stand with your feet hip-width apart.
Bend forward with your knees bent. Place
your hands on your thighs above the knees
for leverage. Lean the weight of your torso
into your hands.

2. Exhale forcefully from your mouth. Close
your mouth and bring your chin to your throat. Hold the
exhalation and pull your abdomen back toward the
spine and up toward the solar plexus.

3. Hold for 2 seconds, then rhythmically pump the
abdominal muscles in and out with a pull-in, release
motion 5 or more times.

4. Before the lack of oxygen becomes uncomfortable, relax the abdominals and inhale slowly. Return to an upright position.

YOGA OBSERVATION

What It Does: Yoga Observation practices *svadhyaya* (the understanding of self), which is part of niyama, one of the eight limbs of yoga as described in Patanjali's *Yoga Sutras* (see Chapter 1). Yoga Observation is the first step to Yoga Relaxation; it entails recognizing stress.

How to Do It:

1. Sit straight in a chair with your legs together and feet flat on the floor. Alternatively, you can sit on the floor in a seated meditation pose, such as Easy Pose (page 74) or Half Lotus Pose (page 77), or lie down in Supported Relaxation Pose (page 128). Be sure that you're comfortable and relaxed in whichever position you choose.

2. Be the observer, looking for stress within your body. Notice without judgment. How does the stress feel? Are you clenching your jaw? Do you have a knot in your stomach? Are you holding your breath? Is your breathing shallow and fast? When you recognize

that you're holding tension, fatigue, or pain in a particular area, try to relax that area.

3. Calmly take note of the flow of your thoughts. Is your mind restless? Do you have negative thoughts and suggestions? Quiet your mind by focusing on your breath. Center your attention on the tip of your nose. Observe the coolness of the air as it flows into your nostrils, and the warmth of the air as it flows out. Focus your attention on your breath. If your mind wanders, simply bring it back to the breath as it flows in and out of your nostrils. Be in the moment.

4. Now replace your negative thoughts with positive suggestions, such as uplifting words, affirmations, thoughts, and prayers. Breathe in love, light, energy, and healing to every cell of your body. Breathe out all negativity, darkness, tension, and fatigue. Rest your body and mind for as long as you like.

chapter 3

Yoga Relaxation and Breathing

Would you like to remain calm, alert, and focused, even as a storm of stress rages around you? You may be one of the millions of people around the globe who have been deeply troubled by shocking global or personal events, and you may be searching for ways to restore a sense of calm and balance to your life. With the relaxation and breathing techniques that follow, you'll tap into yourself and find inner balance as you gain strength and stability. At one time or another we all face chaotic events beyond our control, but we can learn to counter their effects. Yoga practice is a great way to do just that.

Daily life is full of challenging and sometimes stressful moments. Many of us deal with the pressures of two-career households, long work hours, and a shifting economic landscape. It's no wonder we're in the midst of a stress epidemic. The American Institute of Stress has determined that stress lurks behind nearly 90 percent of visits to the doctor. Stress has been linked to all of the leading causes of death, including heart and lung diseases, cirrhosis of the liver, cancer, accidents, and suicide. Research has also confirmed the role of stress in many serious health problems, from depression to insomnia. But don't let the numbers get you down. You can learn to manage and beat stress with regular practice of these relaxation and breathing techniques.

Stress is an inevitable part of life. We usually think of stress as negative—something that knots the stomach, brings shortness of breath, and challenges our immune system. However, certain types of stress are actually good for you. There's the positive stress that helps us to win a race, or that creates sexual tension or inspires us. The magic of yoga is its power to release the negative stress that can cause us harm.

The Stress Response

Stress results from the way we react to a situation, not from the situation itself. It's our reaction to the event that determines its effect on our physical and mental health. For example, if we perceive a situation as dangerous or threatening, we'll experience anxiety and fear. This fearful response generates a fight-or-flight physiological reaction.

Our body's autonomic nervous system is divided into two parts, the sympathetic system—identified with the fight-or-flight response—and the parasympathetic—which counteracts the physiological effects of the sympathetic. Our sympathetic nervous system energizes and prepares us to either flee or engage in battle by releasing stress hormones such as adrenaline. These hormones sharpen perception and reaction, dilating our pupils to allow more light in (to help us see better); increasing our breathing, heart rate, and blood pressure (to maximize blood flow to our limbs); and stopping digestion.

Although the threatening situations have changed, our physiologic reaction to danger is much the same as early man's. Obviously modern negative stressors generally aren't life-or-death situations, but our bodies respond just as cavemen's bodies did when faced with a saber-toothed tiger. When our fight-or-flight response is evoked daily by life's annoying hassles, such as being stuck in traffic or waiting in line at the supermarket, or by more serious life events, such as a death in the family or a contentious divorce, it takes a toll on our health. Our sympathetic nervous system becomes overloaded, often producing chronic muscle tension (especially in the shoulders, neck, and jaw), elevated heart rate and blood pressure, and digestive problems. Left unattended, this can result in chronic illness, pain, and disease.

We can release chronic muscle tension and the other symptoms of negative stress by practicing yoga relaxation and breathing techniques. Performing yoga's relaxation poses and deep breathing turns off the fight-or-flight response and turns on the parasympathetic nervous system, known as the relaxation response. This slows our heartbeat, decreases our blood pressure and respiration, lowers our stress hormone levels, and brings our body back into a healthier balance.

Three Yoga Steps to Relaxation

You can elicit the relaxation response in three easy steps, with yoga practices that help you recognize the stress, release the tension, and breathe deeply. The complete Yoga Relaxation and Breathing Practice Plan follows this section, but first, here's how and why it works.

1. RECOGNIZING THE STRESS

The first step in reversing negative stress is to recognize it. Be aware of what your body is feeling. This is the perfect opportunity to practice the understanding of self, or *svadhyaya*. Be the observer and look for places where stress accumulates within your body (see Yoga Observation, page 29). It makes sense to identify where stress resides in your body, because once you know, you can do something about it.

2. RELEASING THE TENSION

The second step in reversing negative stress is to release the tension. As soon as you become aware of negative stress, stop what you're doing and release it from your body. You can do a few seated yoga tension-relieving poses at your desk or wherever you might be sitting (see the 7-Step Yoga Relaxation Sequence, page 44).

Yoga poses and self-massage are powerful tools to relieve stress and tension. You can easily do any number of poses at your desk, including Seated Head Tap, Seated Shoulder-and-Arm Tap, and Face Massage. As discussed in Chapter 1, *do-in* and self-acupressure can help to relieve and prevent tension and tightness, promote relaxation, and increase the circulation of prana.

Regular yoga asana practice, including vinyasa yoga (see Chapter 5, "Yoga Movement Meditation"), restorative yoga (see Chapter 6, "Restorative Yoga"), and wellness yoga (see Chapter 7, "Yoga for Emotional Wellness"), will also relieve and prevent tension and negative stress.

3. BREATHING DEEPLY

The third step in reversing negative stress is to breathe deeply. Now that you've done some tension-relieving poses, you're ready to slow your breathing down. Yoga deep breathing is a natural tranquilizer for the mind and body. When we're under stress, we hold our bellies rigid and our breathing is shallow. This may deprive the brain, muscles, and vital organs of oxygen. You can change your breathing pattern from tension-producing to relaxation-enhancing by practicing yoga deep abdominal breathing.

By shifting your awareness to your breath and away from upsetting thoughts, you shift your body into relaxation mode. Research indicates that breathing slowly and deeply sends a message to the body and mind that all is well, thereby interrupting the stress cycle.

Take a 1-minute vacation from work with the routine outlined in the Yoga Relaxation and Breathing Practice Plan. You can practice the art and science of *pranayama* (yoga breathing) lying down in Modified Relaxation Pose (see page 24) or sitting up in Easy Pose with Chin Lock (page 58), with techniques including Complete Breath, Alternate-Nostril Breathing, and Cooling Breath, all described in the section "Yoga Breathing *(Pranayama),*" later in this chapter.

Once you become familiar with yoga breathing, follow your pranayama practice with yoga meditation (see Chapter 4, "Yoga Meditation and Mantra"), which has been shown to elicit the relaxation response.

Yoga Breathing Basics

Breathing is something that many of us take for granted, yet it's one of the few autonomic functions we can control consciously. Breathing is an essential part of our survival; it supports all of our basic physiological processes and strongly influences mind, body, and spirit. We can live for a few weeks without food and a few days without water, but for only a few minutes without breath.

Pranayama is one of the eight essential limbs of the Tree of Yoga described in Patanjali's *Yoga Sutras*. In Sanskrit, *yama* means restraint or control. Pranayama seeks to harness and control the breath to direct, circulate, and store *prana* (life-force energy) in the body, to facilitate spiritual enlightenment and reach a higher consciousness.

Yoga masters believe that by slowing down the breath, and thereby slowing down the heartbeat, we may enjoy longevity and perfect health. Regular pranayama practice is a wise investment. With yoga breathing, you may build a supply of life-force energy from which you can draw during times of stress.

Shallow breathing (or even holding the breath) is a typical response to negative stress. In shallow breathing, you are taking air into the chest only, rather than the abdomen, and utilizing only the upper lobes of the lungs. In contrast, with yoga deep breathing you first breathe into the lower abdomen, then the rib cage, and then the upper chest. Utilizing all three areas of the lungs during yoga deep breathing will increase your lung capacity over time and will supply more oxygen for the trillions of cells in your body. You'll also enjoy increased energy, vitality, and life force, and a calm mind.

Deep breathing may be difficult to master at first. My students often find it helpful to visualize the mechanics of deep breathing. The organs and muscles of respiration include the diaphragm—a large, dome-shaped muscle that separates the lungs and heart from the stomach and other abdominal organs—the twelve pairs of ribs, the intercostal muscles between the ribs, the abdominal muscles, a pair of lungs, and the heart. With deep inhalation, your diaphragm presses downward to make more space for the air coming in, your abdomen expands, then your ribs and chest widen to make room for your expanding lungs. On exhalation, your diaphragm rises, pushing the air back out, as your chest, lungs, ribs, and then your abdomen contract.

If you're just beginning pranayama practice, you may find yoga deep breathing easier when you're lying down. That way you don't have to contend with the challenge of maintaining a stable, seated posture while learning pranayama. Begin practicing Complete Breath lying down in Modified Relaxation Pose or Supported Relaxation Pose. Once you're comfortable practicing pranayama lying down—without strain, dizziness, or shortness of breath—you're ready to try a seated pose. Begin your seated pranayama practice with Complete Breath, Easy Pose with Chin Lock, Alternate-Nostril

Breathing, and Cooling Breath. Gate Pose will help you prepare for deep breathing by stretching the intercostal muscles and sides of the body.

Before You Start

- If you have any physical limitations, such as asthma or heart disease, consult your physician before beginning yoga breathing exercises.
- If you're just beginning a yoga breathing practice, comfortably and gradually work up to the recommended frequency and duration of these pranayama exercises. Respect your own abilities.
- You should never experience strain, dizziness, or shortness of breath while practicing pranayama. If any of these symptoms occur, stop immediately. Try a less challenging yoga breathing exercise. If symptoms persist, see your physician.

Yoga Relaxation and Breathing Practice Plan

After practicing the Yoga Basics from Chapter 2 for 1 week, begin this Yoga Relaxation and Breathing practice. Be aware that it may take you more than 4 weeks to do this routine comfortably, depending on your physical condition. If you feel comfortable and confident doing the poses in Weeks 1 and 2, proceed to Week 3, then Week 4. Otherwise, stay with Weeks 1 and 2 until you feel strong enough to continue.

Week 1

Practice Schedule: Practice for 20 to 30 minutes, 3 days a week.

Yoga Observation: Practice seated Yoga Observation (see page 29).

7-Step Yoga Relaxation Sequence: Choose 3 of the following for each practice session:

Seated Head Tap

Face Massage

Seated Head-and-Neck Tilt

Seated Shoulder-and-Arm Tap

Seated Stretch and Yawn

Tighten-and-Release Pose

Progressive Relaxation

Yoga Breathing:

Gate Pose

Complete Breath, lying down in Modified Relaxation Pose or
  Supported Relaxation Pose

Week 2

Practice Schedule: Practice for 20 to 30 minutes, 3 or 4 days a week.

Yoga Observation: Practice seated Yoga Observation.

7-Step Yoga Relaxation Sequence: Choose 4 of the following for each practice session:

Seated Head Tap

Face Massage

Seated Head-and-Neck Tilt

Seated Shoulder-and-Arm Tap

Seated Stretch and Yawn

Tighten-and-Release Pose

Progressive Relaxation

Yoga Breathing:

Gate Pose

Complete Breath, sitting up

Week 3

Practice Schedule: Practice for 30 minutes, 4 days a week.

Yoga Observation: Practice seated Yoga Observation.

7-Step Yoga Relaxation Sequence: Perform the entire sequence in each practice session.

Seated Head Tap

Face Massage

Seated Head-and-Neck Tilt

Seated Shoulder-and-Arm Tap

Seated Stretch and Yawn

Tighten-and-Release Pose

Progressive Relaxation

Yoga Breathing:

Gate Pose

Alternate-Nostril Breathing

Cooling Breath

Week 4

Practice Schedule: Practice for 30 to 40 minutes, 4 days a week.

Yoga Observation: Practice seated Yoga Observation.

7-Step Yoga Relaxation Sequence: Perform the entire sequence in each practice session.

Seated Head Tap

Face Massage

Seated Head-and-Neck Tilt

Seated Shoulder-and-Arm Tap

Seated Stretch and Yawn

Tighten-and-Release Pose

Progressive Relaxation

Yoga Breathing:

Gate Pose

Alternate-Nostril Breathing

Easy Pose with Chin Lock

The 7-Step Yoga Relaxation Sequence

1. SEATED HEAD TAP

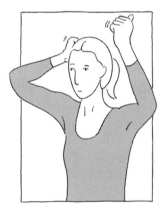

What It Does: Practicing *do-in* in Seated Head Tap helps to release tension and tightness in the head and neck, promotes relaxation, and increases the circulation of prana. This exercise also helps relieve and prevent tension headaches and improves concentration.

How to Do It:

1. Sit straight in a chair with your legs together and feet flat on the floor.

2. Gently and lightly tap all around your head with loosely closed fists. As you tap, take slow, deep breaths.

3. Tap for approximately 10 seconds.

2. FACE MASSAGE

What It Does: Practicing *do-in* and self-acupressure in Face Massage is very helpful for relieving sinus pain as well as chronic tension in the face and jaw.

How to Do It:

1. Sit straight in a chair with your legs together and feet flat on the floor. Before you begin, observe how your face feels. Does your jaw feel tense? Is your face cold? Do you have sinus pain?

2. Moving your fingertips in slow, circular motions, massage your temples, around your hairline, up and down the sides of your nose, in front of your ears, behind your ears and the back of your neck. As you massage, take slow, deep, relaxing breaths.

3. With your fingertips, massage your jaw muscles with firm pressure. Open and close your mouth to find your jaw muscles. As you massage, be sure to continue your relaxed breathing.

4. With the pads of your fingers gently press underneath your cheekbones.

5. Now close your eyes and observe how your face feels after your massage. Does it feel warmer? More awake? Tingling? Has your jaw tension dissolved?

3. SEATED HEAD-AND-NECK TILT

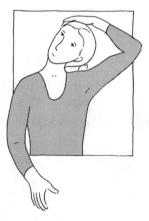

What It Does: Doing Seated Head-and-Neck Tilt releases tension, fatigue, and pain in the head and neck and relieves negative stress.

How to Do It:

1. Sit straight in a chair with your legs together and feet flat on the floor.

2. Inhale, then exhale as you tilt your head to the left toward your left shoulder. Lightly place your left hand on

your head; allow the weight of the hand to gently increase the stretch in the right side of your neck.

3. Take several slow, deep breaths as you relax and stretch the muscles down the right side of your neck, for about 30 seconds.

4. Remove your hand and slowly lift your head to center. Observe the difference in the way the right and left sides of the neck feel.

5. Repeat on the other side.

4. SEATED SHOULDER-AND-ARM TAP

What It Does: Practicing *do-in* in Seated Shoulder-and-Arm Tap helps to relieve and prevent tension and tightness in the neck, shoulders, and arms.

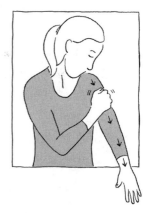

How to Do It:

1. Sit straight in a chair with your legs together and feet flat on the floor.

2. With loosely closed fists, gently and lightly tap from the top of your shoulder, down your arm to your hand.

3. Repeat three times on each arm.

5. SEATED STRETCH AND YAWN

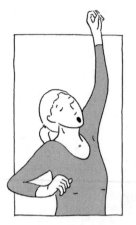

What It Does: The most natural release of tension, fatigue, and stress is to stretch and yawn. Doing Seated Stretch and Yawn releases tension and fatigue in the upper body and relieves negative stress.

How to Do It:

1. With a slow, deep inhalation, raise your arms above your head. Exhale and relax your shoulders down from your ears.

2. Take a deep breath and stretch your left arm up toward the ceiling. Squeeze your mouth and eyes shut, and yawn. Keep stretching the left arm up, while your right arm remains relaxed and your right elbow slightly bent. Exhale and relax the left arm.

3. Take a deep breath as you stretch your right arm up toward the ceiling. Squeeze your mouth and eyes shut, and yawn. Keep stretching the right arm up, while your left arm remains relaxed and your left elbow slightly bent. Exhale and release the right arm down to your side.

4. Repeat on each side.

5. Now observe the sensation that follows. That's what it feels like to release tension from your face and shoulders!

6. TIGHTEN-AND-RELEASE POSE

What It Does: Tighten-and-Release Pose gathers up all the negative stress and tension in the body, holds it, then releases it.

How to Do It:

1. Lie on your back on a mat on the floor. While in-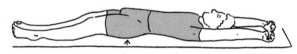
haling, raise your arms above your head and clench your fists. Tighten your buttocks and lift your hips up, while pushing your heels down. Squeeze your mouth and eyes shut, and tense your face, your arms, your hands, your legs, and your feet. *Hold the tension for 5 seconds.*

2. Exhale as you release the tension and relax your feet, your legs, your hands, your arms, and your face. Feel all of the tension drain right out of your muscles, flowing out your hands and feet.

3. Observe the sensation that follows.

7. PROGRESSIVE RELAXATION

What It Does: With Progressive Relaxation we focus sequentially on relaxing each individual body part, beginning with the feet and working up to the head.

How to Do It:

1. Sit straight in a chair with your legs together and feet flat on the floor, or lie down in Supported Relaxation Pose (see page 128). Be sure that you're comfortable and relaxed in this position.

2. Now relax each part of your body, beginning with your feet and working up to your head. Begin by centering your attention on your feet and toes. Inhale and suggest to the feet and toes to relax. Exhale and observe your toes and feet relaxing. Feel the sensation of them melting into the floor.

3. Repeat the three Progressive Relaxation steps, Attention, Positive Suggestion, and Observation, with each individual body part, including your ankles, calves, knees, thighs, and pelvis, noticing and releasing areas of tension. Continue with your upper body, including your abdomen, back, chest, arms, head, and face, noticing and releasing areas of tension.

4. With each exhalation, allow the weight of your bones to sink

toward the floor. Scan your body, noting any muscular tension or pain. Now, with each exhalation, surrender your muscles to the pull of gravity, sinking further into the floor.

5. Relax all efforts and rest in the healing stillness for as long as you wish.

Yoga Breathing *(Pranayama)*

GATE POSE *(PARIGHASANA)*

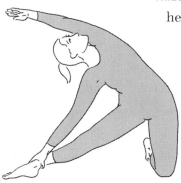

What It Does: The Gate Pose side bend will help you prepare for deep breathing by stretching the intercostal muscles, the muscles that connect the ribs. Use a folded blanket under your supporting knee, if necessary.

How to Do It:

1. Kneel on the floor with your spine in an upright position. If kneeling is painful, place a folded blanket under your knees. If you still experience pain or discomfort, stop immediately.

2. Now straighten your right leg out to the side, with the right foot as flat on the floor as possible and the right knee facing the ceiling. The left knee remains directly below the left hip.

3. Inhale and stretch both arms out to the sides, with palms facing the floor. Exhale and reach up with your left arm, then bend at the waist to the right, placing your right hand on your lower right leg. Look up under your left arm toward the ceiling.

4. Hold for 3 to 5 breaths. Stretch and expand the left side of your rib cage with each inhalation and exhalation.

5. Inhale and lift your left arm overhead while bringing your spine back to center. Exhale and stretch both arms out to the sides. Bring your right leg back to kneeling position.

6. Repeat on the other side.

7. Observe the sensation that follows. Does your breathing feel fuller, deeper?

COMPLETE BREATH (PRANAYAMA)

What It Does: Complete Breath is a classic pranayama technique used during relaxation, but it can be done anywhere, at any time. Practice Complete Breath during times of stress to focus, center, and calm yourself. It is called Complete Breath because it integrates the lower, middle, and upper parts of your lungs. This will increase your lung capacity as well as strengthen your diaphragm, chest, and intercostal muscles.

How to Do It:

1. If you're just beginning pranayama practice, it may be easier to learn Complete Breath lying down in Modified Relaxation Pose (see page 24) or in Supported Relaxation Pose (see page 128). When you're comfortable practicing this exercise lying down, try it sitting in a chair with your legs together and feet flat on the floor, or in a seated pose, such as Easy Pose (see page 74).

2. Gently place both of your hands, fingertips touching, on your abdomen, below the belly button. You want to feel the action of your abdomen as you inhale and exhale.

3. Exhale the air from your lungs completely through your nose. To a total count of 4, smoothly inhale through your nose and feel your fingertips rise as you breathe into your belly (count 1), expand your ribs, filling the middle part of the lungs with air (count 2), and finally draw air into your upper chest, lifting the breastbone (counts 3 and 4). Hold the breath for a moment, feeling the base, middle, and upper parts of the lungs completely expanded.

4. To a total count of 8, slowly exhale through your nose. In a smooth stream of breath, exhale from the upper chest (counts 1 and 2), then from the ribs and middle part of the lungs (counts 3, 4, and 5), and finally from the base of the lungs, feeling your fingertips fall as your belly draws in with the exhalation (counts 6, 7, and 8). This completes 1 round of Complete Breath.

5. Repeat a few rounds of Complete Breath in joyous serenity.

ALTERNATE-NOSTRIL BREATHING
(NADHI SHODHANA)

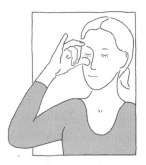

What It Does: Alternate-Nostril Breathing, one of the best-known pranayama techniques, helps balance mind, body, and spirit. Practicing Alternate-Nostril Breathing is a natural tranquilizer, as it calms the nervous system, relieves tension and negative stress, and quiets the mind. It teaches us control of our breathing through the right and left nostrils, and it is also an excellent preparation for meditation. You're ready for this exercise when you feel comfortable and strong doing breathing exercises lying on the floor.

How to Do It:

1. Sit straight in a chair with your legs together and feet flat on the floor, or sit on the floor in a seated yoga position, such as Easy Pose (see page 74) or Half Lotus Pose (see page 77).

2. Close your eyes and bring your attention to your breath. Quietly observe the breath for a few moments.

3. Draw the second and third fingers of your right hand to the center of your palm, then cover your right nostril with your right thumb.

4. Exhale all air from your lungs through your left nostril. Using a Complete Breath inhalation, smoothly inhale through your left nostril, to a total count of 4: breathe into your belly (count 1), expand your ribs, filling the middle part of the lungs with air (count 2), and finally bring air into your upper chest, lifting the breastbone (counts 3 and 4). Feel the lower, middle, and upper parts of the lungs completely expanded.

5. Use your right ring finger and thumb to gently pinch both nostrils closed. Hold the breath for a count of 4.

6. Lift the right thumb and, in a smooth stream of breath, exhale

slowly through the right nostril to the count of 8: exhale from the upper chest (counts 1 and 2), then the ribs and middle part of the lungs (counts 3, 4, and 5), and finally the base of the lungs, as your belly pulls in (counts 6, 7, and 8).

7. Using a Complete Breath inhalation, smoothly inhale through your right nostril, to a total count of 4. Gently press and hold both nostrils closed with your right ring finger and thumb. Hold the breath for a count of 4. Lift the ring finger and, in a smooth stream of breath, exhale slowly through the left nostril to a count of 8. This finishes 1 round of Alternate-Nostril Breathing.

8. Repeat a complete round up to 5 times.

9. When you finish Alternate-Nostril Breathing, sit quietly and observe the sensations that follow. Do you feel calmer, more centered, more in touch with your body, breath, and mind?

COOLING BREATH (SHITALI)

What It Does: This exercise cools the body on a hot day and cools down overheated emotions.

How to Do It:

1. Sit straight in a chair with your legs together and feet flat on

the floor, or sit on the floor in a seated yoga position, such as Easy Pose (see page 74) or Half Lotus Pose (see page 77).

2. Close your eyes and bring your attention to your breath. Quietly observe the breath for a few moments. Once you feel centered and focused, begin Cooling Breath.

3. Open your mouth and roll your tongue into a tube shape. If you can't roll your tongue, raise the sides of your tongue with your fingers.

4. Inhale smoothly though the tunnel, as if you're sipping through a straw. As you inhale, imagine breathing in prana and light.

5. Then unroll your tongue and close your mouth, while exhaling

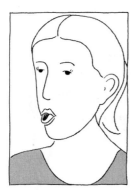

smoothly through your nose. As you exhale, imagine you're breathing out all impurities and darkness of the body, mind, and spirit.

6. Repeat 10 times.

EASY POSE WITH CHIN LOCK
(SUKHASANA JALANDHARA BANDHA)

What It Does: Bandhas, or muscular locks, are used during yoga postures to lock in and regulate prana, thereby preventing its escape from the body. Incorporating *jalandhara bandha,* or "chin lock," into your breathing and meditation poses will increase the storage and circulation of healing prana in your body. It will

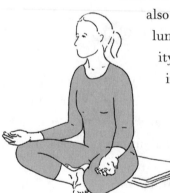

also stretch and open your upper chest and lungs, helping to increase your lung capacity. It is an excellent preparation for meditation. Practice this more advanced posture when you feel comfortable and strong doing breathing exercises lying on the floor.

How to Do It:

1. Sit on the floor, on the edge of a folded blanket. Cross your legs. For this posture, the spine is straight and the knees are lower than the top of the pelvis. If your back is rounded, or your knees are higher than your pelvis, add a second blanket.

2. Place your hands on your knees, palms turned up. Lift your chest upward just slightly, raising the top of your sternum toward your chin. Lower your chin gently toward your chest.

3. Close your eyes and bring your attention to your breath. Quietly observe your breath for a few moments. Once you feel centered and focused, practice several rounds of Complete Breath, described earlier in this chapter. Then return to quietly observing your normal breathing for a few moments. Continue this breathing cycle for 1 to 3 minutes.

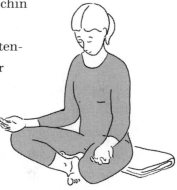

4. As you hold the posture, be sure not to strain your neck. If your neck muscles begin to feel tired, bring your head up into simple Easy Pose.

5. Sit quietly and observe the effect the chin lock had on your breathing. Do you feel calmer, more centered, more in touch with your body, breath, and mind?

chapter 4

Yoga Meditation and Mantra

Twenty-first-century existence, with its multitasking lifestyles, business travel, and sometimes overwhelming stimulation, often creates negative stress. What can you do about it? Learn to meditate! Yoga meditation can help you calm your inner world to better deal with the frantic outer world. Use meditation as a break from the nonstop stimulation that creates anxiety, worry, and stress and you'll quiet and relax the body, mind, and spirit.

Meditation is a yoga technique with a long history as a stress-management tool. Researchers have been studying meditation and its effects for more than thirty-five years, and their results indicate that meditation reduces bodily stress and helps treat many stress-related problems, including heart disease, high blood pressure, depression, anxiety, sleep disorders, headaches, psoriasis, and chronic pain.

According to findings published in *Stroke*, a journal of the American Heart Association, learning to relax and reduce stress through the practice of Transcendental Meditation (TM) may reduce atherosclerosis and the risk of heart attack and stroke. Another study showed that an 8-week, meditation-based stress-reduction program for highly stressed medical and premedical students significantly reduced anxiety and depression and increased empathy.

Meditation is the continuation of the Three Yoga Steps to Relaxation, discussed in the previous chapter. Practicing yoga meditation turns off the fight-or-flight stress response and turns on the parasympathetic nervous system's relaxation response. This slows our heartbeat, decreases our blood pressure and respiration rate, lowers our stress hormone levels, and helps counter the cumulative effects of stress.

Dr. Herbert Benson, author and the director of the Mind/Body Medical Institute at Harvard Medical School, coined the phrase "relaxation response." Dr. Benson's research found that focusing on repeating a word, sound, prayer, phrase, or exercise has a calming effect on the body. This focused repetition of a word, sound, prayer, or phrase is a hallmark of yoga meditation using a mantra. The focused repetition of an exercise is considered a type of movement meditation and is found in vinyasa yoga (see Chapter 5, "Yoga Movement Meditation").

Meditation History

Meditation as well as yoga dates back to the ancient Vedas, sacred Hindu scriptures first recorded around 2500 B.C.E. The Rig Veda and the Upanishads—two of the most ancient texts—are hymns and scriptures of ancient Hindu yoga philosophy. Of the eight limbs of the Tree of Yoga, described by the sage Patanjali in the second century B.C.E., three focus on meditation, namely pratyahara, the withdrawal of the senses for meditation; dharana, concentration for meditation; and dhyana, which includes meditation practice itself.

In the twenty-first century, we are the beneficiaries of the wisdom gained by the flower children of the 1960s, the generation that pioneered the modern exploration of consciousness in the West. Although curiosity and/or hallucinogenic drugs may have initiated their search, some of these early experimenters subsequently focused on meditation and yoga for realizing the divine and, to use the phrase that Aldous Huxley borrowed from William Blake, open the doors of perception.

Ram Dass (born Richard Alpert), hippie guru, author, and former Harvard psychologist, may be one of the most influential spiritual teachers of his generation. He is perhaps best known for the experiments with LSD in the early 1960s that led to his dismissal from the faculty at Harvard, along with countercultural icon and activist Timothy Leary. But his far greater gift has been his long dedication to teaching yoga and meditation to millions. As Ram Dass has taught, practicing meditation will allow us to "be here now" and live in the present moment. There's nothing better for your health than a meditation break.

Choosing a Meditation Style

Over millennia, many styles of yoga meditation practice have evolved, each providing a different path to the same goal—enlightenment. As you search for an approach that's right for you, remember that although many meditation styles are part of a spiritual tradition, they are techniques, not theology.

There are basically two kinds of meditation: meditation that promotes concentration and meditation that promotes mindful awareness. The former, dharana, involves focusing on an object, such as the breath, a mantra, or a candle flame, and away from your anxious thoughts. When you notice your attention has strayed, you bring your attention back to the meditation object. Practice the meditations outlined in the Yoga Meditation Practice Plan (see page 70) to alleviate the negative stress and stimulation in your life that create anxiety, worry, and turmoil. Soon you will feel and radiate a new-found optimism and sense of well-being.

Mindful awareness meditation trains practitioners to detach from and observe their emotions. *Vipassana*, or insight meditation, is a Buddhist practice of mindful awareness. It originated in India and was taught by the Buddha, who was himself a yoga master. Practicing the Mindfulness Meditation described on page 83 will nurture introspection, serenity, and cosmic connectedness, and help develop a life of wisdom and compassion.

Good Vibrations

Mantra is a powerful technique you can use during your yoga meditation. It is the practice of repeating sacred words, phrases, or sound vibrations, which become the focus of concentration during meditation. Mantras can be spoken aloud, sung, chanted, hummed, thought, or written. A mantra can also be used as a tool to invoke spiritual power; to heal and cleanse the body, mind, and spirit; and ultimately to realize samadhi, enlightenment or perfect bliss. Mantras are common to many spiritual traditions, beliefs, and cultures, including Hinduism, Buddhism, Christianity, Judaism, and Sufism.

Eastern-style mantras became known in the Western world with the popularization of Transcendental Meditation in the 1960s. In TM, the meditator receives a personal mantra from his or her guru, and then repeats it mentally for 15 to 20 minutes twice a day. There are hundreds of medical studies documenting TM's many benefits, including deep relaxation, lowered blood pressure, and decreased risk of heart disease.

Fortunately, you don't need a guru to begin to enjoy the benefits of using a mantra in your meditation practice. You can create your own mantra with any word or sound that has a spiritual meaning for you. According to nada yoga, the yoga of sound, finding a mantra that resonates with your body's natural vibration is as simple as finding a word—in Sanskrit or English—that appeals to you.

Sanskrit sounds and words are often employed as mantras because they resonate in specific chakras (the body's energy centers) and energize the body to higher states of consciousness. For example, the word *om* is thought to be the sound of the universe. *Om* is considered to be the universal, sacred, perfect, and supreme mantra, and is one of the most recognized mantras in the West. In addition to a single sound, mantras can take the form of a sacred word, phrase, or prayer. As you practice the meditation exercises that follow, try using different mantras to see what resonates for you. Here are some suggestions:

- *Peace*
- *Love*
- *Shalom* ("Peace" in Hebrew. Pronounced *shah-loam*.)
- *Om* (Pronounced *ah-oh-m*, or *aum*.)
- *Om shanthi, shanthi, shanthi* ("All is peace, peace, peace." Pronounced *aum shahn-tee, shahn-tee, shahn-tee*.)
- *So hum* ("I am that. That which is immortal and everlasting.")

Repeat your mantra in sync with your breathing. You need not voice your mantra; silent or mental recitation is considered to be a powerful form of mantra practice as well. For example, to use the mantra *so hum*, inhale, silently saying *so* to yourself, then exhale, saying *hum*. (See "Om Meditation," page 84.)

Chanting can vibrate with the frequency of love, tune in to the divine, and connect to the highest level of awareness. It can also deepen meditation, calm the mind, remove anxiety and worries, open the heart, and even create an altered state of consciousness or spiritual ecstasy.

In India, holy songs are chanted and sung in a *kirtan*, or ecstatic devotional singing. Simple melodies are repeated many times, often for hours, to achieve spiritual awareness and union with the divine. In the 1960s, Bhagavan Das (born Michael Riggs), a California native, brought kirtan to the West from India. He's perhaps best known for originating the phrase Ram Dass would later immortalize, "Be here now." Today, Bhagavan Das and other ecstatic devotional singers, such as Krishna Das and Jai Uttal, lead formal kirtan sessions at concerts, retreats, workshops, and yoga centers, connecting new generations to this powerfully spiritual experience. You can reap the benefits of chanting by practicing the Bhramari Hum described on page 85.

Three Meditation Guidelines

To relieve stress through meditation, follow these three guidelines: Preparation, Posture, and Practice.

1. PREPARATION

Prepare your body, mind, and attention for meditation and reverse negative stress by following the Three Yoga Steps to Relaxation detailed in Chapter 3: recognizing the stress, releasing the tension, and breathing deeply.

2. POSTURE

Although full Lotus Pose is commonly associated with meditation, it may not be comfortable for you. Lotus Pose is a natural resting pose for the people of India. If done correctly, it perfectly aligns the body and spine for meditation. In following the Yoga Meditation Practice Plan, try Half Lotus Pose in Week 2 of practice, and as you grow stronger and more flexible, try the full Lotus Pose. Beginners may be most comfortable in Easy Pose. Other, more challenging yoga meditation poses to try are Kneeling Pose and Hero Pose. (All are described later in this chapter.)

If it's painful to hold a yoga sitting pose for the duration of your meditation practice, you may want to sit in a chair, with your head, neck, and spine straight and in alignment. If sitting in a chair becomes painful after 10 minutes, try meditating lying down in Supported Relaxation Pose (see page 128). Few people can hold a meditation pose with perfect ease right from the start, but with consistent practice you will become strong and flexible enough to hold the pose for the full length of your practice.

3. PRACTICE

Be consistent with your meditation practice. Try to set aside a specific time of day to meditate—every day, if possible. Yogis consider sunrise and sunset to be auspicious times of day to meditate; the important thing is that you choose a time that works best for you, and stick with it. Remember, this time is for you, to prevent and treat negative stress, to relax and rejuvenate your mind and body.

You may also want to designate a special place to meditate, whether it's at your desk or in a cozy corner in your home. A quiet space where you're not likely to be disturbed is best. Before beginning meditation, many practitioners enjoy lighting a candle or incense, or diffusing essential oils.

If you can't arrange a consistent time and place to meditate, try including meditation in your daily activities. You can practice movement meditation with vinyasa yoga, while walking mindfully or when waiting on line (see Chapter 5, "Yoga Movement Meditation").

Before You Start

If you're suffering from stress-related problems, be sure to consult your physician, in addition to practicing this yoga relaxation and meditation program.

Yoga Meditation Practice Plan

After practicing the Yoga Relaxation and Breathing routines found in Chapter 3, begin this Yoga Meditation Practice. Be aware that it may take you more than 4 weeks to do this routine comfortably. If you feel comfortable and confident doing the poses in Weeks 1 and 2, proceed to Week 3, then Week 4. Otherwise, stay with Weeks 1 and 2 until you feel strong enough to continue.

Prepare your body, mind, and attention for meditation and reverse negative stress by following the Three Yoga Steps to Relaxation outlined in the previous chapter: recognizing the stress, releasing the tension, and breathing deeply. Now that you've done tension-relieving poses and pranayama, you're ready to meditate. Practicing these yoga meditation poses will help you grow strong enough to sit in a pose for the duration of your meditation.

Week 1

Practice Schedule: Practice for 30 to 40 minutes, 3 days a week.

Yoga Observation: Practice seated Yoga Observation (see page 29).

7-Step Yoga Relaxation Sequence: Do all 7 poses during each practice session (see page 44).

Seated Head Tap

Face Massage

Seated Head-and-Neck Tilt

Seated Shoulder-and-Arm Tap

Seated Stretch and Yawn

Tighten-and-Release Pose

Progressive Relaxation

Yoga Breathing and Meditation:

Complete Breath (see page 52) in Easy Pose Relaxation Meditation, lying down in Supported Relaxation Pose (see page 128)

Week 2

Practice Schedule: Practice for 30 to 40 minutes, 4 days a week.

Yoga Observation: Practice seated Yoga Observation.

7-Step Yoga Relaxation Sequence: Do all 7 poses during each practice session.

Seated Head Tap

Face Massage

Seated Head-and-Neck Tilt

Seated Shoulder-and-Arm Tap

Seated Stretch and Yawn

Tighten-and-Release Pose

Progressive Relaxation

Yoga Breathing and Meditation:

Alternate-Nostril Breathing (see page 54) in Easy Pose or Half Lotus Pose

Flower Power Meditation, seated in chair

Week 3

Practice Schedule: Practice for 30 to 40 minutes, 4 or 5 days a week.

Yoga Observation: Practice seated Yoga Observation.

Yoga Relaxation:

Tighten-and-Release Pose

Progressive Relaxation

Bound Lotus and Variation

Yoga Breathing and Meditation:

Easy Pose with Chin Lock (see page 58)

Om Meditation in Easy Pose or Kneeling Pose

Week 4

Practice Schedule: Practice for 40 minutes, 4 or 5 days a week.

Yoga Observation: Practice seated Yoga Observation.

Yoga Relaxation:

Tighten-and-Release Pose

Progressive Relaxation

Bound Lotus and Variation

Yoga Breathing and Meditation:

Bhramari Hum in Easy Pose or Half Lotus Pose

Mindfulness Meditation in Easy Pose, Hero Pose, Half Lotus
    Pose, or Lotus Pose

Yoga Meditation Postures

EASY POSE *(SUKHASANA)*

What It Does: This restful pose increases flexibility in the hips, legs, and ankles. It is used for
meditation, pranayama, and the cultiva-
tion of calmness.

How to Do It:

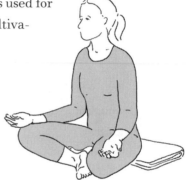

1. Sit on the floor, on the edge
of a folded blanket. Cross your
legs. For this posture, the spine is
straight and the knees are lower
than the top of the pelvis. If your
back is rounded, or your knees are higher
than your pelvis, add a second blanket.

2. Place your hands on your knees, palms turned up. Close your
eyes and bring your attention to your breath.

3. As your flexibility increases, dispense with the blanket and sit
directly on the floor, centered on your sit bones.

KNEELING POSE (VAJRASANA)

What It Does: Kneeling Pose is commonly practiced by Zen Buddhist monks, as well as yogis, during meditation. To protect your knees, kneel on a folded blanket or pillow.

How to Do It:

1. Place a folded blanket or a pillow under your knees. Kneel with your shins parallel and the tops of your feet extended and your toes pointing straight back. Proper alignment of your shins and feet will prevent knee strain.

2. Sit on your heels. Rest your palms on your thighs. Keep your spine in an upright position.

3. Hold for 3 breaths. When you can hold the pose comfortably, practice pranayama or meditation.

HERO POSE (VIRASANA)

What It Does: Hero Pose stretches the quadriceps muscles, knees, ankles, and tops of the feet. Begin by sitting on a folded blanket, a book, or a block, then gradually lower the prop (use a thinner book, then a blanket) until you can comfortably sit on the floor.

How to Do It:

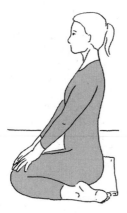

1. Kneel on the floor with your shins parallel and the tops of your feet extended and your toes pointing straight back. Keep your spine in an upright position. Proper alignment of your shins and feet will prevent knee strain. Sit on a folded blanket or a telephone book positioned between your feet. Rest your palms on your knees. Feel the stretch at the tops of your thighs, and in your ankles and feet.

2. When you're ready, lower or remove the prop. Do not force this position! If your knees, ankles, or feet feel strain or pain, you're not ready.

3. Hold for 3 breaths. When you can hold the pose comfortably, practice pranayama or a meditation technique (choose one below).

4. To come out of the pose, return to kneeling.

HALF LOTUS POSE
(ARDHA PADMASANA)

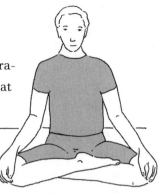

What It Does: Half Lotus Pose is preparation for a classic meditation posture that teaches proper leg, ankle, and foot alignment and restores flexibility to the hips and legs. If your hips are very tight, your knees will stick up in the air when you attempt Half Lotus. With practice, your knees will come closer to the floor. Forcing this pose may cause knee strain, so don't force it. Instead, practice Easy Pose for a week or more before trying Half Lotus Pose again.

How to Do It:

1. Sit on the floor in a cross-legged position. Gently grasp your right foot and carefully place it on top of your left thigh as close to your hip as possible. The sole of the foot faces upward. Do not force this position! If your right knee feels strain or pain, or is sticking up in the air, you're not ready to do this pose.

2. Sit up straight, lifting your sternum, palms resting on your knees. Hold for a few seconds, breathing comfortably.

3. Gently release the right foot back to cross-legged position. Repeat pose with your left foot. When you can hold the pose comfortably, practice pranayama or a meditation technique (choose one below).

LOTUS POSE *(PADMASANA)*

What It Does: Lotus Pose is a classic meditation posture that teaches proper leg, ankle, and foot alignment and restores flexibility to the hips and legs. If your hips are very tight, your knees will stick up in the air when you attempt Lotus. With practice, your knees will eventually come closer to the floor. Forcing this pose may result in knee strain, so don't force it. Instead, prepare for full Lotus Pose by practicing Easy Pose and Half Lotus Pose. A folded blanket placed under the hips can help your legs and hips rotate into proper alignment.

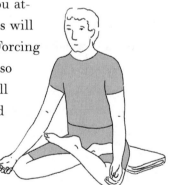

How to Do It:

1. Sit on the floor, with a folded blanket under your hips and your legs extended. Bend your right leg and gently grasp your right foot. Turn the sole of your right foot to face you, and carefully place your foot on top of your left thigh as close to your hip as possible. Do not force this position! If you feel strain or pain in your knee, or it sticks up in the air, stop immediately. You're not ready to do this pose.

2. Bend your left leg and gently grasp your left foot. Turn the sole of your left foot upward, facing you, and lift your foot an inch or two. If this causes discomfort, stop! Do not continue. If you feel you can continue safely, then gradually and carefully place your right foot on your left thigh as close as possible to your hip. Again, do not force this position!

3. Sit up straight, lifting your sternum. Bring thumb and index fingers together and rest your hands, palms up, on your knees. Hold for 3 breaths. When you can hold the pose comfortably, practice pranayama or a meditation technique (choose one below).

4. Gently release your feet from your thighs. Repeat Lotus Pose with the leg positions reversed.

BOUND LOTUS AND VARIATION (*YOGA MUDRA*)

What It Does: Bound Lotus and Variation releases tension and negative stress in the body and is an excellent preparation for meditation.

How to Do It:

1. Begin by sitting in Easy Pose, Half Lotus, or full Lotus Pose. Clasp your hands behind your back and interlock your fingers.

2. Inhale, lifting your sternum toward the ceiling. Straighten your elbows and gently squeeze your shoulder blades together. Raise your chin toward the ceiling.

3. Exhale, slowly lowering your forehead to the floor, with your arms extended behind you, hands clasped and fingers interlocked. Hold for 2 breaths.

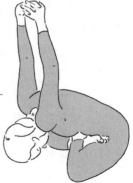

4. Inhale and slowly return to upright position. Exhale and release your clasped hands. Rest your hands on your knees. Observe the release of tension and stress in your shoulders and arms.

Yoga Meditation

RELAXATION MEDITATION

What It Does: In Relaxation Meditation, a sound, word, phrase, or prayer is repeated, creating a calming effect on the body. Experiment until you find a word or sound, such as *peace, relax,* or *love,* that resonates for you.

How to Do It:

1. Sit straight in a chair with your legs together and feet flat on the floor; or assume a seated meditation posture such as Easy Pose (see page 74) or Half Lotus Pose (see page 77); or lie down in Supported Relaxation Pose (see page 128). You should be comfortable and relaxed in the position you choose.

2. Close your eyes and bring your attention to your breath. Quietly observe the breath for a few moments. As you breathe out, silently mouth the word or phrase you've chosen.

3. Continue for 10 to 20 minutes, breathing in, then breathing out, silently mouthing your word.

4. If distracting thoughts or mental images arise, don't fight them or dwell on them, simply focus again on your breath and your word.

5. Sit quietly for a few minutes, first with your eyes closed, then with your eyes open.

FLOWER POWER MEDITATION

What It Does: Flower Power Meditation guides us to "be here now"—to live in the present moment, where peace, equanimity, and the Divinity reside.

How to Do It:

1. Sit straight in a chair with your legs together and feet flat on the floor; or assume a seated meditation pose such as Easy Pose (see page 74) or Half Lotus Pose (see page 77); or lie down in Supported Relaxation Pose (see page 128). You should be comfortable and relaxed.

2. Close your eyes and bring your attention to your breath. Quietly observe the breath flowing in and out at the tip of your nose. As you breathe in, silently say to yourself, "Breathing in," and as you breathe out, silently say, "Breathing out."

3. Continue for 10 to 20 minutes, focusing on the tip of your nose and following your breath, silently mouthing, "Breathing in," then "Breathing out," over and over again.

4. If distracting thoughts or mental images arise, just bring your attention back to your breath. Don't fight the thoughts or dwell on them, simply return to the breath. Imagine that each distracting thought is like the petal of a flower, such as a daisy, and your breath is in the center of the daisy. When a distracting thought brings your attention away from the breath, from the center of the flower, you've traveled out on a petal. When you notice your distracting thought, simply bring your focus back to the center of the daisy—your breath.

5. Sit quietly for a few minutes. Observe the sense of peace and well-being you feel after your meditation. You will begin to connect to that place behind your thoughts, where perfect bliss, or samadhi, resides.

MINDFULNESS MEDITATION

What It Does: Mindfulness Meditation is calm observation of the mind. It nurtures introspection, serenity, and cosmic connectedness, and helps develop a life of wisdom and compassion.

How to Do It:

1. Sit straight in a chair with your legs together and feet flat on

the floor; or assume a seated meditation pose such as Easy Pose (see page 74) or Half Lotus Pose (see page 77); or lie down in Supported Relaxation Pose (see page 128). You should be comfortable and relaxed.

2. Close your eyes and with awareness observe your thoughts and feelings as they go through your mind. Don't become involved with the passing thoughts, simply allow them to come and go. Observe each thought in a detached manner, and let it go.

3. After a while, your thoughts will come to a complete stop and you will enter the silence of the mind. Meditate in the silence for 10 to 20 minutes. It is here that healing begins.

4. Sit quietly for a few minutes. Observe the sense of peace and well-being you feel after your meditation.

OM MEDITATION

What It Does: The Sanskrit word *om* (pronounced *ah-oh-m*, or *aum*) is thought to be the sound of the universe. *Om* is considered to be the universal, sacred, perfect, and supreme mantra. It is believed that stress, tension, and worry are alleviated and the mind becomes calm through meditation with the mantra *om*. Other mantras to try are *om shanthi, shanthi, shanthi* ("All is peace, peace, peace"), pronounced *aum shahn-tee, shahn-tee, shahn-tee,* and *so hum,* ("I am that. That which is immortal and everlasting").

How to Do It:

1. Sit straight in a chair with your legs together and feet flat on the floor; or assume a seated meditation pose such as Easy Pose (see page 74) or Kneeling Pose (see page 75); or lie down in Supported Relaxation Pose (see page 128). You should be comfortable and relaxed.

2. Close your eyes and bring your attention to your breath. Quietly observe the breath for a few moments. As you breathe in, silently mouth the word *om,* and again as you breathe out, say *om* silently. If you're practicing with the mantra *so hum,* breathe in as you mouth *so,* and out as you mouth *hum.*

3. Continue for 10 to 20 minutes, silently saying your mantra. Be aware of the gaps between your breaths. As your mind becomes still, you'll notice gaps in your thoughts as well as your breath.

4. Sit quietly for a few minutes, just be-ing in the present moment.

BHRAMARI HUM

What It Does: Mantras can be hummed, as well as spoken and sung. *Bhramari* is the humming sound of a bee, a soft *eee* sound.

How to Do It:

1. Sit straight in a chair with your legs together and feet flat on the floor; or assume a seated meditation pose such as Easy Pose (see page 74) or Half Lotus Pose (see page 77). You should be comfortable and relaxed.

2. Smoothly inhale through your nose to the count of 5: breathe into your belly (count 1); then into your ribs, filling the middle part of the lungs with air (counts 2 and 3); and finally draw air up into the upper chest, lifting the breastbone (counts 4 and 5). Feel the base, middle, and upper part of the lungs expanded completely.

3. Exhale slowly through your nose to the count of 10, using your throat to make a soft *eee* humming sound: exhale from your upper chest (counts 1, 2, and 3), then from your ribs and the middle part of the lungs (counts 4, 5, and 6), and finally from the base of the lungs, as your belly pulls in (counts 7, 8, 9, and 10). Remain focused on the sound.

4. Repeat breathing in to the count of 5 and out to the count of 10, up to 5 times.

5. Sit quietly and observe the sensations that follow. You should feel calmer, more centered, more in touch with your body, breath, and mind.

chapter 5

Yoga Movement Meditation

Would you like to reduce stress; improve your flexibility, strength, and cardiovascular fitness; and find inner peace at the same time? You can achieve all that and more with the Yoga Movement Meditation practice that follows. Yoga Movement Meditation combines vinyasa (a continuous flow of yoga poses), such as Sun Salutation, with meditation. This powerfully effective combination of yoga and meditation makes the most of your workout time.

The Yoga Movement Meditation Workouts are excellent fitness routines for everyone, regardless of size, shape, age, or fitness level. These routines are also helpful if you're having difficulty finding time to both meditate and participate in a cardiovascular fitness program consistently.

I also recommend this practice for those who have difficulty with sitting meditation. Many highly stressed people find it difficult, if not impossible, to slow their breathing down and remain calm long enough to practice sitting meditation. The Yoga Movement Meditation Workouts are the perfect solution to this common dilemma.

Movement meditation, also known as focused or mindful exercise, quiets the mind and relieves tension through a combination of gentle exercises and meditation. As discussed in Chapter 4, repeating a word, phrase, or sound has a calming effect on the body, producing what is known as the relaxation response. The same is true of repeating certain kinds of exercise.

Yoga's Aerobic Benefits

In ashtanga-style yoga we perform vinyasas, a series of poses that follow one another in a continuous flow. *Ashtanga vinyasa* features the same postures as hatha yoga, except these poses are linked together, in synchrony with the breath. The result is a safe cardiovascular workout that perfectly blends flexibility, strength, and aerobic conditioning.

According to medical experts, 30 minutes of moderate activity over the course of a day, 3 times a week, will reward you with a long list of benefits, including reduced risk of developing heart disease or dying prematurely. Moderate aerobic activities include brisk walking, stationary cycling, jogging, and ashtanga vinyasa yoga. One of the misconceptions about yoga is that it doesn't provide a cardiovascular workout. On the contrary, a vigorous ashtanga vinyasa yoga practice such as the Sun Salutation can be just as effective as many aerobic activities in improving cardiovascular health, boosting endorphins—the feel-good hormones—and promoting strength, flexibility, mental clarity, and self-esteem.

Medical experts have found that regular aerobic exercise by itself reduces stress hormone levels, anxiety, and negative stress. However, research has shown that combining rhythmic, repetitive aerobic exercise (such as Sun Salutation practice) with meditation increases those stress-relief benefits and activates the relaxation response. Studies have also shown that meditation improves muscular efficiency. For example, runners who incorporated meditation into their training were able to run farther and longer. They also reported experiencing a "runner's high" in the first mile, an endorphin surge that is usually thought to occur in the third or fourth mile.

Asanas and Meditation

You can practice yoga asanas, or poses, without meditation, and still experience stress relief. That's because each pose in itself can become a type of meditation. With asana practice, the body is the focus of concentration. Ideally, the focus is on moving in synchrony with your breath while maintaining an inner calm as you practice challenging physical postures.

Oftentimes, we get caught up in goal-oriented thoughts as we practice asanas. We focus on precision of movement or technique, rather than on cultivating meditation. This is especially true for beginners. If you're a beginning yoga student, you may be too involved in trying to remember the specifics of each pose and the sequence of poses to add meditation to the mix. Be patient. As you become more proficient and confident you'll be able to incorporate meditation into the Sun Salutation routine.

As discussed in Chapter 4, there are two basic meditation techniques: those that promote concentration and those that promote mindful awareness. The former involve focusing on an object of meditation, such as the breath, a mantra, or a candle flame. Mindful awareness is calm observation of the mind.

Combining Breath, Asanas, Mantra, and Attention

You can combine yoga meditation with Sun Salutation asanas in the following three ways:

1. UJJAYI PRANAYAMA AND SUN SALUTATION

Ujjayi breathing is a classic yoga breathing technique (see Chapter 2) that can be joined with Sun Salutation asanas to promote concentration. Focusing on the breath while practicing the series of poses calms the mind. Breath becomes the object of meditation and replaces anxious thoughts. Practice ujjayi breathing with Sun Salutation in the routine that follows.

2. ADDING A MANTRA

Ujjayi breathing can be combined with mantra and Sun Salutation asanas to promote deeper states of meditation. As discussed in Chapter 4, mantra is the practice of using repeated sacred words, phrases, or sound vibrations as a focus of concentration during meditation. Popular mantras include *om, peace,* and *so hum.* You can create your own mantra with any word or sound that has a spiritual meaning for you. Experiment until you find one that resonates for you.

To combine mantra with ujjayi breathing, first focus your attention on the inhalation and exhalation of your ujjayi breath during your Sun Salutation practice. When you've connected your breath and posture flow, add a silent mantra, such as *om*. With each ujjayi inhalation and exhalation, mouth the word *om*. If distracting thoughts or mental images occur, don't fight them or dwell on them, simply return to repeating your mantra.

3. ADDING MINDFUL AWARENESS

We can also integrate mindful awareness with ujjayi breathing and Sun Salutation asanas. This combination of meditative components can be a powerful tool for expanding consciousness. With mindful awareness, you simply observe your thoughts and feelings as they pass through your mind. Don't become involved with these thoughts; simply allow them to come and go.

To combine mindful awareness with ujjayi breathing, first focus your attention on the inhalation and exhalation of your ujjayi breath during your Sun Salutation practice. Now cultivate a state of moment-to-moment mindfulness by becoming aware of the gaps *between* your ujjayi breaths. In a detached manner, observe any thoughts that may arise, and let them go. After a while, your thoughts will stop and your mind will become calm.

Yoga Meditation and Walking

If you would like to increase the time you devote to meditation, you can combine a yoga meditation technique with your daily activities, such as walking, washing dishes, or standing in line at the bank or supermarket.

Walking combined with yoga meditation is a superlative way to alleviate stress and derive important cardiovascular benefits. In walking meditation, we combine walking with ujjayi breathing and mantra, just as we did with Sun Salutation asanas.

Begin your walking meditation by focusing your attention on the inhalation and exhalation of your ujjayi breath as you walk. As you inhale and exhale, follow the breath as it flows in and out through the nose. Once you've established the connection between the rhythm of your breath and your steps, add a mantra, such as *om*. With each ujjayi inhalation and exhalation, say *om*. If distracting thoughts or mental images occur, don't fight them or dwell on them, simply return to repeating your mantra.

Another walking meditation technique involves counting the number of steps you take as you breathe in and out. You will soon discover the natural pattern of your breathing. Your lungs may be comfortable taking 2 steps as you breathe in and 2 steps as you breathe out—what I call a 2/2 step pattern. Or you may find that you are comfortable with a 2/3 step pattern—taking 2 steps as you breathe in and 3 steps as you breathe out.

Incorporate a mantra that matches your pace. For instance, in a 2/2 step pattern, silently say *so* with your ujjayi inhalation, and say *hum* with your exhalation. After practicing for a while, you may want to increase the number of steps you take as you inhale, to improve the cardiovascular benefits of your walk. If you've been practicing a 2-step pattern, increase to a 3-step (3/3) pattern, taking 3 steps when you inhale and 3 when you exhale.

When you finish your walking meditation, stand quietly and observe the calmness you're feeling.

Before You Start

- Always consult your physician before beginning a new exercise program.
- If you're just beginning a fitness program, comfortably and gradually work up to the recommended frequency and duration of exercise.
- Perform the vinyasas slowly, according to your own abilities. You should never be in pain or breathless. Pay attention to your body's signals of overexertion, such as pounding in your chest, dizziness, faintness, profuse sweating, or an inability to carry on a normal conversation. If any of these symptoms occur, slow down. If the symptoms persist, see your doctor.
- Do not practice movement meditation in a challenging environment, or while driving a moving vehicle.

Your 4-Week Yoga Movement Meditation Workouts

You can begin the Yoga Movement Meditation Workout after practicing the Yoga Meditation routines found in Chapter 4 for 4 weeks.

As you progress from the Beginner to the Maintenance workout over a period of 2 months and beyond, you'll build your yoga practice up from 30 to 60 minutes a day, 3 to 5 days a week. For additional stress-relief benefits, you can incorporate the Restorative Yoga Workout (see Chapter 6) and Wellness Yoga Workout (see Chapter 7) into your practice.

Yoga Movement Meditation Workout Plans

1. BEGINNER YOGA MOVEMENT MEDITATION WORKOUT

After practicing the Yoga Meditation routines found in Chapter 4 for 4 weeks, beginners should start with this workout. After you've finished this 4-week plan, you can proceed to the Intermediate Yoga Movement Meditation Workout. Be aware that it may take you more than 4 weeks to do this routine comfortably. Feel free to take as much time as you need before progressing to Intermediate practice.

Weeks 1 and 2

Practice Schedule: Practice for 30 to 40 minutes, 3 or 4 days a week.

Yoga Observation: Practice seated Yoga Observation (see page 29).

Warm Up:

7-Step Yoga Relaxation Sequence (see page 44)

Ujjayi Pranayama (see page 26)

Sun Salutation: Perform 4 to 6 repetitions of Sun Salutation without Ujjayi Pranayama.

Cool Down: Supported Relaxation Pose (see page 128).

Weeks 3 and 4

Practice Schedule: Practice for 40 minutes, 4 days a week.

Yoga Observation: Practice seated Yoga Observation.

Warm Up:

7-Step Yoga Relaxation Sequence

Sun Salutation: Perform 6 repetitions of Sun Salutation with Ujjayi Pranayama (see discussion earlier in this chapter).

Cool Down: Supported Relaxation Pose.

2. INTERMEDIATE YOGA MOVEMENT MEDITATION WORKOUT

After practicing the Beginner workout for 4 weeks or more, begin this Intermediate workout. Be aware that it may take you more than

4 weeks to do this routine comfortably. Feel free to take as much time as you need before progressing to Maintenance practice.

Weeks 1 and 2

Practice Schedule: Practice for 50 minutes, 4 days a week.

Yoga Observation: Practice seated Yoga Observation.

Warm Up:

7-Step Yoga Relaxation Sequence

Bound Lotus and Variation (see page 80).

Sun Salutation: Perform 6 repetitions of Sun Salutation with Ujjayi Pranayama and mantra (see "Adding a Mantra" earlier in this chapter).

Walking Meditation (optional): Do walking meditation with mantra for 10 to 15 minutes, 3 days a week.

Cool Down: Supported Relaxation Pose.

Weeks 3 and 4

Practice Schedule: Practice for 50 minutes, 5 days a week.

Yoga Observation: Practice seated Yoga Observation.

Warm Up:

7-Step Yoga Relaxation Sequence

Bound Lotus and Variation

Sun Salutation: Perform 6 to 8 repetitions of Sun Salutation with Ujjayi Pranayama and mindful awareness (see "Adding Mindful Awareness" section earlier in this chapter).

Walking Meditation (optional): Do walking, mantra, and steps meditation (see page 93) for 10 to 15 minutes, 3 days a week.

Cool Down: Supported Relaxation Pose.

3. MAINTENANCE YOGA MOVEMENT MEDITATION WORKOUT

Congratulations! At this point, you've mastered the Beginner and Intermediate workouts. I'm sure you're looking and feeling great. Do the Maintenance Yoga Movement Meditation Workout to continue to build and maintain your stress-relief, cardiovascular fitness, and flexibility benefits.

Week 1 and Beyond

Practice Schedule: Practice for 50 to 60 minutes, 5 days a week.

Warm Up:

7-Step Yoga Relaxation Sequence

Bound Lotus and Variation

Sun Salutation: Perform 6 to 8 repetitions of Sun Salutation with Ujjayi Pranayama and mantra or mindful awareness.

Walking Meditation (optional): Do walking, mantra, and steps meditation for 10 to 15 minutes, 3 days a week.

Cool Down: Choose one of the following Yoga Breathing and Meditation routines (see Chapter 4):

Complete Breath in Easy Pose

Relaxation Meditation, lying down in Supported Relaxation Pose

OR

Alternate-Nostril Breathing in Easy Pose or Half Lotus Pose

Flower Power Meditation, seated in a chair

OR

Easy Pose with Chin Lock

Om Meditation in Easy Pose or Kneeling Pose

OR

Bhramari Hum in Easy Pose or Half Lotus Pose

Mindfulness Meditation in Easy Pose, Hero Pose, Half Lotus Pose, or Lotus Pose

SUN SALUTATION *(SURYA NAMASKAR)*
WITH MEDITATION

What It Is: This ancient, classic yoga routine is traditionally done at sunrise, but can of course be practiced at any time of day. It is a complete workout for body and mind.

How to Do It: With each inhalation and exhalation, adding Ujjayi Pranayama (Beginner workout, Weeks 3 and 4), plus mantra (Intermediate, Weeks 1 and 2) or mindful awareness (Intermediate, Weeks 3 and 4) as you progress through the plan.

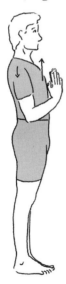

1. Mountain Pose *(Tadasana):* Stand with your feet together, legs straight, kneecaps tightened and pulled up, weight distributed evenly, and hands in prayer position over your heart center. Tilt your pelvis under, abdomen pulled in and shoulders relaxed and down, away from your ears. Lift your sternum toward the ceiling. This pose teaches correct posture.

2. Standing Backbend: Inhale and raise your arms in a V overhead. Tighten your buttock muscles firmly to protect your lower back, lift your chest toward the ceiling, and bend backward. Pause for 3 seconds.

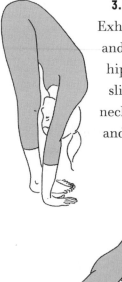

3. Standing Forward Bend *(Uttanasana)*: Exhale, extending your arms forward, and fold your torso forward from the hips, abdomen in. Bend your knees slightly. Relax your face, head, neck, and shoulders toward the floor and lower your chest to your thighs. Place your hands on the floor, fingers in line with your toes.

4. Left Lunge *(Anjaneyasana)*: Inhale, bending both knees and keeping your palms flat beside your feet. Step your right foot back, bringing your right knee to the floor. Stretch your chin up toward the ceiling. Your left knee should be directly over your left ankle (i.e., shin perpendicular to the floor).

5. Plank Pose *(Dandasana)*: Exhale, bringing your left leg back to join the right, and extend your arms, as you would to begin a push-up. Keep your body straight, legs and arms extended and head in line with spine. Pull your stomach in. Hold for 1 or 2 breaths.

6. Modified Plank Pose *(Modified Chaturanga Dandasana)*: Exhale, bending and lowering your knees, chest, and chin to the floor. Hips are up, abdomen is in. This pose is similar to a modified women's push-up. Keep your elbows close to your body. Or, if this is too difficult, go from Plank Pose to placing the body

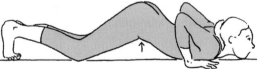

flat, face down on the floor. Then go into a modified women's push-up position.

7. Cobra Pose (*Bhujangasana*): Inhale, raising your forehead, chin, and chest while arching your spine. Hips are on the floor. Elbows should be slightly bent and close to the body. Shoulders are pressed down and away from the ears. Tilt your pelvis under for lower-back protection. Pause for several breaths.

8. Downward-Facing Dog (*Adho Mukha Svanasana*): Exhale, lifting your hips up and back, as you turn your body into an upside-down V. Keep your arms and legs straight and press your heels toward the floor. Draw your shoulders down and away from your ears.

9. Right Lunge (*Anjaneyasana*): Inhale, lunging your right foot forward between your two hands, toes in line with fingers. Look up, chin raised, palms flat, left knee on the floor.

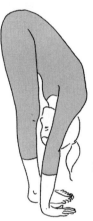

10. Standing Forward Bend (*Uttanasana*): Exhale, pushing off with the toes of your left foot to bring the left foot forward to join the right. Upper body is folded forward from the hips, knees are slightly bent, hands are on either side of the feet.

11. Standing Backbend: Inhale, raising yourself upright, keeping your back straight, your arms extended overhead, and your knees slightly bent. Exhale and tighten your buttocks. Inhale, keeping your head between your arms; lift the sternum toward the ceiling and arch your spine backward. Pause for 3 seconds.

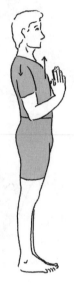

12. Mountain Pose *(Tadasana)*: Exhale; return to an upright position and bring your palms together. Take a few breaths, breathing in light and energy, exhaling tension and fatigue.

Repeat Steps 2 through 12 on the opposite leg, bringing the left leg back for Step 4, then forward for Step 9, for a complete cycle.

chapter 6

Restorative Yoga

Don't despair if time is short. You can rest, relax, and revitalize in minutes with the Restorative Yoga Workout that follows. Restorative yoga is the practice of active relaxation to relieve stress, restore health, replenish vitality, and live in the present moment. The asanas featured in this routine are therapeutic variations of the basic Relaxation Pose (Savasana) combined with yoga breathing (pranayama). Using props, blankets, and bolsters to support the body and help maximize stretch, restorative poses can induce deep states of relaxation, improve sleep and immune function, reduce tension and fatigue, lower blood pressure, and help relieve pain.

Stressful emotions, such as fear, anger, and depression, and other toxic energies are often manifested in tense muscles. This special type of yoga practice will deeply relax the muscles, releasing stressful memories and toxin buildup from your muscles. Restorative poses also increase circulation, bringing freshly oxygenated blood to the muscles, along with endorphins, the body's natural painkillers.

Yoga Props

In restorative yoga we use props such as blankets, bolsters, blocks, pillows, straps, and chairs to help induce deep states of relaxation. Props help support the body so that you can totally let go. Props also ensure correct alignment and compensate for physical limitations. Using props will help prevent muscle, back, and knee strain due to weakness, lack of flexibility, or balance problems. For example, folded blankets placed beneath the supine body are used for Supported Relaxation Pose, Supported Bridge Pose, and Lying Bound Angle Pose. You can safely assume an inverted position with the support of any wall, as shown in Legs-up-the-Wall Pose.

Yoga and Aromatherapy

Instead of snacking on high-calorie junk food and collapsing on the couch after a stressful day, unwind and relax with restorative poses and the soothing scents of essential oils. A calming ritual of yoga complemented by burning an incense stick, or diffusing essential oils or anointing your body with them, will relieve stress, help you collect your thoughts, and refresh your body, mind, and spirit.

Aromatherapy is an ancient art and science that uses the essential oils of flowers and plants to enhance and balance mental, spiritual, and physical health. The use of essential oils dates back to the ancient Greeks, Egyptians, and people of India, who luxuriated in these precious oils for health and beauty. Today, holistic aromatherapy is commonly used in Europe and India by health practitioners and ayurvedic physicians for stress management and a variety of ailments. It has even established a place among alternative healing therapies in the United States.

Always dilute essential oils before applying them to the skin, and avoid applying them to your eyes, nose, or mouth. To dilute, add 2 drops of essential oil to 1 tablespoon of carrier oil, such as sesame, sweet almond, or jojoba oil. Since essential oils are very concentrated, it is a good idea to test for sensitivity before using a particular oil. To test, apply a little of the diluted essential oil behind your ears and leave it there for 24 hours. If there is no redness or itching, the oil should be safe for you to use. Be sure to keep the oils out of the reach of children.

Ayurvedic Aromatherapy

Ayurveda, the ancient Indian healing system for the mind, body, and spirit, includes aromatherapy for stress relief. Ayurveda is based on the theory of the three *doshas*, or mind-body types, which have their own set of physical, mental, and emotional characteristics; they are *vata* (air), *pitta* (fire), and *kapha* (earth). All people and things possess elements of each dosha, but one or more of the doshas may predominate in your body and behavior. For example, you may be a vata-pitta, pitta-kapha, or vata-kapha. Your unique combination of doshas is your constitution type, or *prakruti*, which establishes your physical, mental, and emotional makeup. An effective way to relieve stress is to identify your dosha, then use specific essential oils to help balance your dosha through the sense of smell.

WHAT'S YOUR DOSHA?

To determine which dosha is most dominant in your body, make a check mark over the individual characteristics (see pages 111–113) that describe you. The category with the most check marks will indicate your dosha. If you have almost the same number of check marks in two or more categories, your body type is a mixture of those two or three doshas. This list of characteristics will give only a rough indication of your dosha. An ayurvedic physician can best determine your dosha body type.

Once you determine your dosha, try using the essential oils in your category to help relieve stress.

BODY TYPE: VATA

Physical Characteristics: Thin, light-boned, angular build; slow to gain weight; dry skin and hair; eats and sleeps erratically; chilly hands and feet; low ratio of muscle to fat; fat accumulates below the navel (prone to potbelly on a lean frame).

Mental and Emotional Characteristics: Quick mind, creates and learns quickly, forgets easily, enthusiastic, imaginative, vivacious. Prone to worry and depression.

Aromatherapy: Benefits from a mixture of warm, sweet, and sour essential oils, such as orange, rose geranium, and clove.

BODY TYPE: PITTA

Physical Characteristics: Medium-size, athletic build; well-proportioned; blond, red, or prematurely gray hair; fair or freckled complexion; warm, ruddy, perspiring skin; good stamina; voracious appetite and tendency to overeat; tends to be warm or hot; sleeps well; eats meals quickly; likely to develop ulcers; gains and loses weight easily; apple shape when overweight.

Mental and Emotional Characteristics: Confident, passionate, articulate, courageous, intelligent, ambitious. Prone to irritability and short temper.

Aromatherapy: Benefits from a mixture of sweet, cool essential oils, such as rose, jasmine, sandalwood, and peppermint.

BODY TYPE: KAPHA

Physical Characteristics: Large, heavy build; wide shoulders; voluptuous or barrel-chested; gains weight easily and has trouble losing it; thick, moist skin and lustrous hair; difficulty with digestion; prone to respiratory illness; excellent stamina; needs more sleep than vata or pitta; eats slowly; pear shape when overweight.

Mental and Emotional Characteristics: Forgiving, affectionate, relaxed, slow and graceful, slow to anger, calm, tolerant. Prone to lethargy and procrastination.

Aromatherapy: Benefits from a mixture of warm, spicy essential oils, such as eucalyptus, clove, and juniper.

According to the ayurvedic and yogic view of aromatherapy, individuals of all doshas will derive stress-relief benefits from using the following essential oils:

Calming Essential Oils: Rose, jasmine, lavender, chamomile, orange, and sandalwood oils all calm and comfort stressed-out bodies, minds, and spirits and promote meditation.

Stimulating Essential Oils: Eucalyptus, peppermint, ginger, clove, rosemary, and sage oils all help stimulate creative thinking, promote understanding, and assist in pranayama.

Mixing Special Aromatherapy Blends

Try blending your choice of soothing essential oils to use before or after your yoga practice to promote a centered calmness and encourage your body, mind, and spirit to relax. You can create an individualized massage oil according to your dosha, a calming oil or a stimulating oil. For example, add approximately 6 drops of calming essential oils, such as chamomile, lavender, or rose, alone or in combination, to 1 ounce of a carrier oil, such as sesame (preferred in Ayurveda), sweet almond, or jojoba oil. Anoint your body at your pulse points, before or after practice.

Aromatherapy During Practice

You can easily incorporate aromatherapy into your yoga practice in several ways.

You can create a fragrant-friendly environment by *diffusing* your favorite calming scents during your yoga practice. Try adding several drops of essential oils, such as orange or jasmine, alone or in combination, to a diffuser, an aromatherapy lamp, or a light bulb ring.

Burning incense is a popular tradition in the practice of yoga and Ayurveda. It is often used for healing, expanding consciousness, purification, and sacred practices. Burning frankincense, myrrh, or sandalwood incense will calm, soothe, and uplift your spirits. This has been part of spiritual practice in many religions for millennia.

The aromas will produce a spiritually uplifting atmosphere for you to practice restorative yoga poses, meditation, and pranayama. For safety, incense sticks should be burned in incense holders; resins can be burned on small pieces of charcoal in metal burners.

Aromatherapy Baths

You can take an aromatic bath to induce deep rest and therapeutic sleep, before or after practice. Add 6 to 10 drops of calming essential oils, such as chamomile, lavender, or rose, alone or in combination, to a comfortably warm bath and gently swirl the water to combine. Or combine 2 drops of essential oil to 1 tablespoon of carrier oil and add the mixture to the bathwater.

Before You Begin

It is always important to consult your physician before beginning any therapeutic program, especially if you are pregnant or have a medical condition. Essential oils should never be ingested, unless intake is supervised by a health care professional.

Restorative Yoga Workout Plan

If your time is limited, the Restorative Yoga Workout can be practiced on its own. You will reap stress-relief benefits even if you have only 10 minutes to do this yoga practice. For maximum stress relief, combine this workout with any of the Yoga Movement Meditation Workouts in Chapter 5. For example, see the combination of the Maintenance Movement Meditation Workout and the Restorative Yoga Workout below.

Be aware that it may take you more than 4 weeks to do this routine comfortably, depending on your physical condition. If you feel comfortable and confident doing the poses in Weeks 1 and 2, proceed to Weeks 3 and 4. Otherwise, stay with Weeks 1 and 2 until you feel strong enough to continue.

Weeks 1 and 2

Practice Schedule: Practice for 10 minutes, 3 days a week, with aromatherapy (optional).

Restorative Poses: Choose 2 from the following:

Legs-up-the-Wall Pose

Supported Relaxation Pose

Supported Bridge Pose

Modified Child's Pose

Weeks 3 and 4

Practice Schedule: Practice for 10 to 15 minutes, 3 times a week, with aromatherapy (optional).

Restorative Poses: Choose 2 from the following:

Bound Angle Sequence

Supported Plough Pose

Supported Seated Angle Pose

Supported Relaxation Pose

Maintenance Movement Meditation and Restorative Yoga Workout

A combination of the Restorative Yoga Workout and the Maintenance Yoga Movement Meditation Workout will act as an ongoing stress reliever while providing cardiovascular-fitness and flexibility benefits.

Week 1 and Beyond

Practice Schedule: Practice for 60 minutes, 5 days a week. On practice days 1, 3, and 5, add Restorative Yoga poses after Sun Salutation (or optional walking meditation).

Warm Up:

7-Step Yoga Relaxation Sequence (see page 44)

Bound Lotus and Variation (see page 80)

Sun Salutation: Perform 6 to 8 repetitions of Sun Salutation with ujjayi breathing and mantra or mindful awareness (see the "Ujjayi Pranayama and Sun Salutation," "Adding a Mantra," and "Adding Mindful Awareness" sections in Chapter 5).

Walking Meditation (optional): Do walking, mantra, and steps meditation (see Chapter 5) for 10 to 15 minutes, 3 days a week.

Restorative Poses: On practice days 1, 3, and 5, do the Restorative Yoga Workout.

Cool Down: Choose a yoga breathing and meditation routine from the Yoga Meditation Practice Plan (see page 70).

Complete Breath in Easy Pose

Relaxation Meditation, lying down in Supported Relaxation Pose

OR

Alternate-Nostril Breathing in Easy Pose or Half Lotus Pose
Flower Power Meditation, seated in chair

OR

Easy Pose with Chin Lock
Om Meditation in Easy Pose or Kneeling Pose

OR

Bhramari Hum in Easy Pose or Half Lotus Pose
Mindfulness Meditation in Easy Pose, Hero Pose, Half Lotus
   Pose, or Lotus Pose

Restorative Yoga Poses

THE BOUND ANGLE SEQUENCE

What It Does: Bound Angle Pose, Bound Angle Variation, and Lying Bound Angle should be practiced one after the other to relieve tension and negative stress, quiet the mind, and rest deeply. Bound Angle Pose and its variations will gently stretch the hips, thighs, knees, and ankles and prepare the body for sitting meditation.

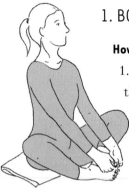

1. BOUND ANGLE POSE *(BADDHA KONASANA)*

How to Do It:

1. Sit on the floor, bend your knees, and bring the soles of your feet together. Sit tall, lifting your sternum toward the ceiling. If your back is rounded, place a folded blanket under your hips.

2. Draw your heels in toward your hips. Place your hands around your feet or your big toes and allow gravity to release your hip joints and pull your knees down toward the floor.

3. Hold the pose for several breaths, breathing comfortably.

4. Continue into Bound Angle Variation.

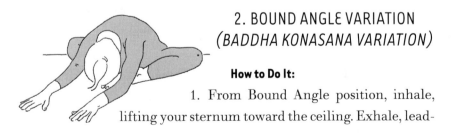

2. BOUND ANGLE VARIATION *(BADDHA KONASANA VARIATION)*

How to Do It:

1. From Bound Angle position, inhale, lifting your sternum toward the ceiling. Exhale, lead-

ing from the sternum and stretching your torso forward, keeping your spine elongated. Extend your arms forward and place your hands on the floor in front of you. Do not force or strain.

2. Inhale and elongate the spine. Exhale, extending the torso farther forward, gradually increasing the stretch. Go only as far as feels comfortable. Hold the pose for several breaths.

3. Slowly sit up in Bound Angle position and continue into Lying Bound Angle.

3. LYING BOUND ANGLE POSE
(SUPTA BADDHA KONASANA)

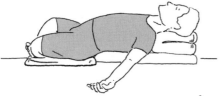

How to Do It:

1. Use a bolster or two folded blankets under your back, a folded blanket under your head, and a folded blanket under your thighs. From Bound Angle position, lie back, keeping the soles of the feet together, until your head is resting on the blankets, with your back, neck,

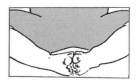

and head fully supported. The arms are in a relaxed T position, palms up.

2. Close your eyes, relax your face, throat, and groin, and take calm breaths through your nose. Rest in this pose for up to 15 minutes.

LEGS-UP-THE-WALL POSE
(MODIFIED VIPARITA KARANI)

What It Does: This is a safe and simple way to get all the benefits of an inversion posture. It improves circulation to the upper body and head and calms the mind.

How to Do It:

1. Sit on the floor beside a wall, with one shoulder as close to the wall as possible. The knees are bent.

2. Swing around and bring both legs up against the wall as you lie back on the floor. Extend your legs straight up the wall with your arms at your sides, keeping your buttocks

against the wall. Breathing comfortably, stay in this position for 1 minute.

3. If your hamstring muscles are stiff and tight, bend your knees a bit. If your lower back, shoulders, and neck are uncomfortable, place a folded blanket or towel beneath them.

4. Come out of the pose by bending your knees, turning to one side, and slowly sitting up. Follow Legs-up-the-Wall with Modified Child's Pose.

MODIFIED CHILD'S POSE
(MODIFIED SALAMBA BALASANA) WITH SELF-MASSAGE

What It Does: Modified Child's Pose with Self-Massage provides deep relaxation and stretching of the back muscles as it relieves back tension, pain, and fatigue. The addition of *do-in* to this pose enhances its healing benefits.

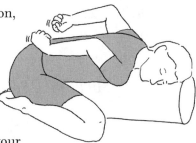

How to Do It:

1. Kneel in front of a bol- ster or folded blankets. Spread your

knees wide, but keep your big toes touching. Put the bolster or folded blankets between your thighs, drawn up to your groin. If sitting on your ankles is uncomfortable, place a pillow under your ankles and feet.

2. Inhale, then exhale slowly and bend forward, lowering your torso to rest on the bolster or blankets. Relax your arms around the support. Turn your face to one side. Relax deeply. Breathe comfortably.

3. Gently tap your lower back and pelvis with lightly closed fists several times.

4. Now relax all efforts. Inhale healing breath into your back. As you exhale, relax your back, visualizing it becoming longer as all tension is released. Continue your visualization as you breathe comfortably.

5. Rest in the pose for as long as you wish. Return to sitting slowly.

SUPPORTED BRIDGE POSE
(SUPPORTED SETU BANDHASANA)

What It Does: Supported Bridge Pose gently opens the chest and upper back, while rejuvenating the body and mind. Use two separate stacks of two or three folded blankets each, or two bolsters, and place them end to end to support the legs, hips, and back. The shoulders, head, and neck should rest comfortably on the floor.

How to Do It:

1. Lie back on the blankets, so that your shoulders, neck, and head are resting comfortably on the floor and your arms are resting by your sides, palms up.

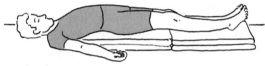

2. Close your eyes and take calm breaths through your nose. Rest in this pose for up to 15 minutes.

3. Come out of the pose by sliding your body backward off the blankets, onto the floor. Roll to your side and pause for a breath or two. Slowly sit up.

SUPPORTED SEATED ANGLE POSE
(SUPPORTED UPAVISTHA KONASANA)

What It Does: Supported Seated Angle Pose gently opens the legs, hips, and pelvis, while revitalizing the body and mind.

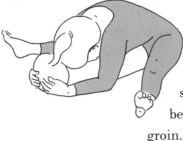

How to Do It:

1. Sit on the floor with a bolster or several folded blankets in front of you. Straighten your legs and spread them apart. Put the bolster between your thighs, drawn up to the groin.

2. Inhale, then exhale slowly and bend forward, lowering your torso to rest on the bolster. Relax your arms around the support. Turn your face to one side or rest your forehead on the blankets. Breathe comfortably and rest in the pose for 5 minutes.

3. Return to sitting slowly.

SUPPORTED PLOUGH POSE (*SUPPORTED HALASANA*)

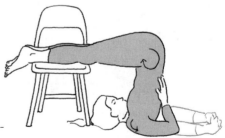

What It Does: This simpler, supported version of Plough Pose promotes mental and physical relaxation and relieves tension and insomnia. Place a chair sideways 8 to 12 inches from your head. Do not proceed with this pose if you feel excessive pressure or pain in the back of the head or neck.

How to Do It:

1. Lie on your back, feet together, hands at sides. Inhale and raise your legs straight up toward the ceiling.

2. Exhale and raise your hips off the floor, using your hands to push off. Place your lower legs on the seat of the chair. Clasp your hands behind your torso and lengthen your arms away from your head. Pull your shoulders down and away from your ears, and rotate your shoulder blades toward your spine.

3. Rotate and press your pelvis under, elongating your spine. Now bend your arms at the elbows and place your hands on your back. The elbows are parallel and close together. Press your shoulders and elbows down as you elongate your spine.

4. Breathe comfortably in this position for up to 1 minute.

5. To come out of the pose, bend both knees to your forehead and bring your hands to the floor. Slowly and with control, bring your hips to the floor. Straighten your legs and lower them.

SUPPORTED RELAXATION POSE
(SUPPORTED SAVASANA)

What It Does: This is the granddaddy of all the restorative poses. Savasana enhances the effectiveness of all the poses, calms the mind and nervous system, and helps relieve back tension.

How to Do It:

1. Lie on your back on a mat on the floor with a folded blanket under your head and neck. You may want to put an additional folded blanket or two under your back and/or cover your eyes with an eye pillow or face cloth.

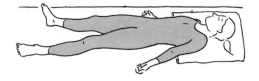

2. Place your feet a comfortable distance apart. Rest your hands at your sides, palms turned upward. Move your shoulders down and away from your ears, and tuck your shoulder blades in toward your spine. If your back feels uncomfortable with your legs straight, bend your knees as much as you need to, to alleviate pain or discomfort. You may feel more comfortable with a folded blanket or pillow beneath your knees.

3. Inhale; exhale, contracting your buttock muscles and pressing the curve out of your lower back. Release and relax completely.

4. Continue to breathe comfortably. With each exhalation, allow the weight of your bones to sink toward the floor. Scan your body, including your spine and your lower back, noting any unnecessary muscular tension. Now, with each exhalation, surrender your muscles to the pull of gravity, sinking further into the floor.

5. Relax all efforts and rest in the healing stillness for as long as you wish. When you're ready to come out of the pose, roll onto one side and use your arms to push yourself up into a seated position.

chapter 7

Yoga for Emotional Wellness

Anxieties over challenging world events and the uncertainties of the times, along with personal problems involving our health, finances, work, or relationships, can create overwhelming stress. These stressors can overload our nervous systems and lead to depression, fatigue, irritability, heightened anxiety, and insomnia.

Yoga can help us to heal and care for ourselves, which in turn enables us to care for others. Yoga teaches us that challenging events bring opportunities for spiritual evolution and healing transformation. Yoga's path guides us as we travel on the cosmic road to emotional wellness, to heal and strengthen our bodies, minds, and spirits. Try the yoga poses that follow to help reduce your anxiety load and restore balance in your life.

Beat the Blues

Everyone experiences the blues once in a while. Mild or moderate depression affects millions of people worldwide, with women twice as likely to be affected as men. Depression is characterized by low energy, loss of interest in life, feelings of hopelessness, and/or sleep disturbances. Depression can be a response to stressful life events, such as divorce or the death of someone close to you, or the result of your genetic makeup, hormonal imbalances, or biochemical abnormalities, such as decreased levels of the neurotransmitter serotonin in the brain.

Yoga practice can be an important part of an antidepression program. Studies have shown that regular aerobic exercise, such as walking, biking, or ashtanga vinyasa yoga, boosts endorphins—the feel-good hormones—and can help prevent and treat depression. To derive the antidepression benefits of aerobic exercise, try the Maintenance Movement Meditation and Wellness Yoga Workout in this chapter, which includes vinyasa Sun Salutation practice.

Inversion poses in particular, such as Half Shoulderstand and Modified Spread-Leg Forward Bend, can help relieve depression by increasing the blood flow to the brain. Preliminary research has indicated that improved blood flow to the brain and endocrine glands enhances the production of feel-good brain chemicals such as seratonin and endorphins.

Yogis have observed that breathing and spinal alignment exercises have a positive effect on the nervous system, mind, and emotions. They've found that practicing backbending postures such as Cobra, Fish, and Bow Poses, coordinated with inhalations, is stimulating and energizing and can counteract lethargy and low moods.

Another asana for your antidepression arsenal is Lion Pose, which releases suppressed emotions and tensions that can lead to depression. The Lion Pose also balances the action of the thyroid, an important endocrine gland (an underactive thyroid can cause depression).

Calm with Yoga

According to the National Institute of Mental Health, anxiety disorders are the most common of all mental illnesses, affecting more than nineteen million Americans each year. Anxiety disorders are characterized by chronic worry, nervousness, irritability, tension, panic, and/or fear. In many cases, anxiety can be so overwhelming that it impairs the individual's ability to function in work and social situations. While prescription medicines can be used to treat anxiety disorders, they also carry the risk of unwanted side effects.

Regular aerobic exercise—including vinyasa yoga—is an all-natural antianxiety treatment that studies have shown is a great outlet for nervous tension. To derive the antianxiety benefits of aerobic exercise, try the Maintenance Movement Meditation and Wellness Yoga Workout in this chapter, which includes Sun Salutation practice.

Yoga balancing poses, such as Modified Tree Pose and Eagle Pose, are an effective way to keep anxiety from getting the better of you. The intense concentration required to balance on one leg prevents anxious thoughts from intruding, and teaches equanimity in challenging situations.

Yoga relaxation and breathing techniques (see Chapter 3) have been used successfully in treating anxiety. Doing Alternate-Nostril Breathing is especially effective in preventing and treating full-blown anxiety attacks. In addition, the relaxation skills learned from regular practice of yoga Progressive Relaxation can be applied in work and social settings, to prevent or alleviate anxiety attacks. These antianxiety benefits are found in the Maintenance Movement Meditation and Wellness Yoga Workout that follows.

Seated and lying twists, such as Half Lord of the Fishes Pose and Crocodile Twist Pose, are powerful anxiety relievers. These poses require concentrating on the breath, which provides an alternative focus of attention and calms anxious thoughts. Forward bends, such as Modified Head-to-Knee Pose, coordinated with exhalations, is calming and relaxing and counteracts nervousness and anxiety.

Sweet Dreams with Yoga

According to the National Sleep Foundation, millions of Americans suffer from sleep problems, and sleep deprivation—reported to affect two-thirds of American adults—is considered one of America's top health problems. Most adults require 8 hours of sleep a night for good health and optimum performance. Yet the majority get considerably less. No doubt the epidemic proportions of this problem stem from our nonstop society, where millions of people trade off quality sleep time for more work time.

Stress, anxiety, and depression are also important causes of sleep disorders, such as insomnia, sleep apnea, restless legs syndrome, and narcolepsy. Insomnia, the most common sleep disorder, is the inability to fall asleep or stay asleep long enough to feel refreshed the next day. Getting good-quality sleep is essential for maintaining and restoring exemplary health. Studies have shown that sleep deprivation depresses the immune system, causes hormonal imbalances, increases the likelihood of accidents, and accelerates the aging process. For these reasons, adequate sleep is considered an essential component of a healthy life.

Before you reach for a sleeping pill and the potentially harmful side effects that come with it, try the Wellness Yoga practice that follows. The combination of sleep-enhancing yoga poses, vinyasa, relaxation, and breathing will help chase away sleepless nights and bring sweet dreams.

Studies have shown that regular aerobic exercise, such as walking combined with meditation or Sun Salutation practice (included in the Maintenance program that begins on page 140), can help promote deep sleep and reduce stress. To tone the nervous system and eliminate emotional and physical stress and tensions that may interfere with sleep, practice Yoga Rock and Roll, Camel Pose, and Modified Head-to-Knee Pose. Before bedtime or while lying awake in bed, practice Progressive Relaxation and Complete Breath while in Relaxation Pose.

Good Bedtime Habits

The sleep-enhancing Wellness Yoga practice, along with the following good bedtime habits, can help you enjoy a good night's sleep.

- **Keep a regular schedule.** Go to bed and wake up at the same time each day. Ayurveda, yoga's sister science, recommends an early bedtime—around 10 P.M.—for optimum-quality sleep.
- **Limit or avoid caffeine, nicotine, and alcohol.** Drinking caffeinated beverages such as coffee and soft drinks during the day can keep you up at night. Drinking alcohol near bedtime interrupts sleep patterns.
- **Create an inviting sleep atmosphere.** Keep your bedroom at a comfortable temperature, neither too hot nor too cold, and free of noise and light.
- **Use your bedroom only for sleep.**
- **Take a warm bath before you go to bed.** Add relaxing essential oils (see Chapter 6) to a bath taken 30 minutes before bedtime.
- **Do vigorous exercise only during the day.** Practice Progressive Relaxation and yoga breathing before going to bed.

Before You Begin

If you're suffering from recurrent, constant, or severe symptoms of depression, anxiety, or insomnia, consult a licensed counselor, psychologist, or psychiatrist for diagnosis and treatment.

Wellness Yoga Workout Plan

If your time is limited, the Wellness Yoga Workout can be practiced on its own. You will reap stress-relief benefits even if you have only 10 minutes to do this yoga practice. For maximum stress relief, combine this workout with any of the Yoga Movement Meditation Workouts in Chapter 5. For example, see the combination of the Maintenance Movement Meditation and Wellness Yoga Workout on page 140.

Be aware that it may take you more than 4 weeks to do this routine comfortably, depending on your physical condition. If you feel comfortable and confident doing the poses in Weeks 1 and 2, proceed to Weeks 3 and 4. Otherwise, stay with Weeks 1 and 2 until you feel strong enough to continue.

Weeks 1 and 2

Practice Schedule: Practice for 10 to 20 minutes, 3 days a week.

Depression-Relief Poses: If you're feeling low, do the following poses:

Modified Spread-Leg Forward Bend

Cobra Pose

Lion Pose

Anxiety-Relief Poses: If you're anxious, do the following poses:

Modified Tree Pose

Crocodile Twist Pose

Alternate-Nostril Breathing (see page 54)

Progressive Relaxation (see page 50)

Insomnia-Relief Poses: If you're suffering from insomnia, do the following poses:

Yoga Rock and Roll

Modified Head-to-Knee Pose

Complete Breath (see page 52) at bedtime

Progressive Relaxation at bedtime

Weeks 3 and 4

Practice Schedule: Practice for 10 to 20 minutes, 3 days a week.

Depression-Relief Poses: If you're feeling low, do the following poses:

Half Shoulderstand

Fish Pose

Bow Pose

Anxiety-Relief Poses: If you're anxious, do the following poses:

Eagle Pose

Half Lord of the Fishes Pose

Modified Head-to-Knee Pose

Alternate-Nostril Breathing

Progressive Relaxation

Insomnia-Relief Poses: If you're suffering from insomnia, do the following poses:

Camel Pose

Modified Head-to-Knee Pose

Complete Breath at bedtime

Progressive Relaxation at bedtime

Maintenance Movement Meditation and Wellness Yoga Workout

A combination of the Wellness Yoga Workout and the Maintenance Yoga Movement Meditation Workout will act as an ongoing stress reliever while promoting emotional wellness, cardiovascular fitness, and flexibility.

Week 1 and Beyond

Practice Schedule: Practice for 60 minutes, 5 days a week. On practice days 1, 3, and 5, add Wellness Yoga poses after Sun Salutation (or optional walking meditation).

Warm Up:

7-Step Yoga Relaxation Sequence (see page 44).

Bound Lotus and Variation (see page 80).

Sun Salutation: Perform 6 to 8 repetitions of Sun Salutation with ujjayi breathing and mantra or mindful awareness (see the "Ujjayi Pranayama and Sun Salutation," "Adding a Mantra," and "Adding Mindful Awareness" sections in Chapter 5).

Walking Meditation (optional): Do walking, mantra, and steps meditation (see Chapter 5) for 10 to 15 minutes, 3 days a week.

Wellness Poses: On practice days 1, 3, and 5, do the Wellness Yoga Workout.

Cool Down: Choose a yoga breathing and meditation routine from the Yoga Meditation Practice Plan (see Chapter 4).

Complete Breath in Easy Pose

Relaxation Meditation, lying down in Supported Relaxation Pose

OR

Alternate-Nostril Breathing in Easy Pose or Half Lotus Pose

Flower Power Meditation, seated in chair

OR

Easy Pose with Chin Lock

Om Meditation in Easy Pose or Kneeling Pose

OR

Bhramari Hum in Easy Pose or Half Lotus Pose

Mindfulness Meditation in Easy Pose, Hero Pose, Half Lotus Pose, or Lotus Pose

Wellness Yoga Poses

MODIFIED SPREAD-LEG FORWARD BEND
(MODIFIED PRASARITA PADA UTTANASANA)

What It Does: This inversion pose increases blood flow to the brain, helping to relieve depression. Using a block will help release and stretch tight hips and hamstrings and prevent lower-back strain. Use an appropriately sized block—one that suits your flexibility needs or limitations. As you grow stronger and more flexible, you can lower the prop (replacing the block with a book, for example), until you can comfortably reach the floor with your hands.

How to Do It:

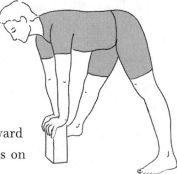

1. Place the block about 1 foot in front of you between your wide-spread legs (your feet should be 3 to 4 feet apart).

2. Inhale, then exhale, folding forward from the hips and placing your hands on the block. Pull your abdomen in.

3. Hang comfortably for 6 to 8 breaths.

4. Come to standing, pulling your abdominals in.

HALF SHOULDERSTAND
(ARDHA SARVANGASANA)

What It Does: This classic inversion pose increases blood flow to the brain, helping to relieve depression. It also tones and strengthens the entire body. This is a simpler version of and preparation for the full shoulderstand, which requires the supervision of a qualified instructor. To protect your neck, practice on a neatly folded towel or blanket, with your shoulders 3 to 4 inches from the folded edge and your head on the floor. You can still reap full shoulderstand benefits by doing this beginner's posture. Always follow with Fish Pose.

How to Do It:

1. Lie on your back, legs extended and feet together, and hands at your sides. Inhale, raising straight legs toward the ceiling.

2. Exhale and raise your hips off the floor, using your hands to push off. Support your pelvis with your hands cupped around your hips, elbows close together. Keep your legs at a 45-degree angle.

3. Hold the pose for 30 to 60 seconds. Breathe comfortably.

4. Bend both knees to your forehead; bring your hands to the floor. Slowly and with control, bring your hips to the floor. Straighten your legs and lower them to the floor. If your back and abdominal muscles are weak, bend your knees to your forehead and lower your bent legs to the floor.

FISH POSE (MATSYASANA)

What It Does: Always do Fish Pose after Half Shoulderstand. It opens the neck and throat area, thereby stimulating the thyroid. The circulation of fresh blood it promotes is naturally stimulating and energizing, and it counteracts lethargy and low moods.

How to Do It:

1. Lie on your back, legs together. Slide your hands, palms down, under your buttocks.

2. Inhale, arch your back, and lift your chest away from the floor, placing your weight on your elbows. Squeeze your shoulder blades together. Roll your head back and lightly touch the mat with the crown of your head.

3. Build up to 2 breaths while holding the position. If your neck feels painful or weak, immediately come out of the position.

COBRA POSE *(BHUJANGASANA)*

What It Does: Cobra Pose stretches and strengthens the back, arms, chest, and shoulders. This pose is stimulating and energizing, and it counteracts lethargy and low moods.

How to Do It:

1. Lie on your stomach with feet together. Place your hands under your shoulders, with your fingers pointing forward. Forehead is resting on the mat. Shoulders are pressed down and away from the ears. Tilt the pelvis under for lower-back protection.

2. Inhale, lifting your forehead, nose, and chin. Slowly raise your chest off the floor and arch your spine, while continuing to keep your shoulders pressed down and your pelvis tilted under. Hips remain on the floor. Elbows should be slightly bent and close to the body. Pause for several breaths.

3. Inhale, then exhale as you lower your body to the mat, leading with your sternum and keeping your shoulders pressed down. When your chest reaches the mat, tuck in your chin, nose, and forehead.

BOW POSE (DHANURASANA)

What It Does: This stimulating pose stretches and tones the abdominal muscles, increases flexibility in the spine, increases stamina, and firms the buttocks.

How to Do It:

1. Lie on your stomach with your forehead on the mat. Reach back and grasp your ankles firmly, keeping your knees hip-width apart. The arms are straight.

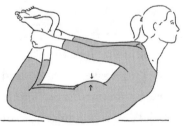

2. Inhale, then exhale, lifting your forehead, nose, and chin. Raise your chest off the floor. To protect your lower back, tighten your buttocks and tuck your pelvis under. Raise your knees off the floor.

3. Inhale, squeezing your shoulder blades together, and lift your breastbone up. Relax your neck.

4. Exhale, releasing the intensity of the stretch slightly, then inhale, lifting your chest and rib cage a little further.

5. Hold for a moment. Exhale and release the stretch slightly, then inhale and lift the chest even higher.

6. Release your hands from your ankles and lie on your stomach. Rest for a moment.

7. Repeat 2 times.

LION POSE *(SIMHASANA)*

What It Does: Lion Pose helps release suppressed emotions and tensions that can cause depression. Practicing this pose can balance the thyroid, an important endocrine gland (an underactive thyroid can cause depression).

How to Do It:

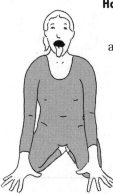

1. Sit on your heels with your knees slightly apart. The fingers are spread open and the hands rest on the knees.

2. Inhale deeply; then, holding the breath slightly, rise off your heels, as if you're a lion about to pounce.

3. Open your mouth and exhale with a *haaa* sound, while sticking out your tongue and opening your eyes wide.

4. Now relax your face and close your eyes. Feel the sensation that follows. Does your face feel warmer, less tense?

MODIFIED TREE POSE
(MODIFIED VRKSASANA)

What It Does: Modified Tree Pose is a standing meditation that promotes mindfulness and calm. It improves balance, strengthens the legs, and increases the flexibility of hips and groin. A belt or strap will help keep your foot from slipping and maintain your hip's open position. As you grow stronger and more confident, dispense with the belt and practice the pose alongside a wall or chair for support.

How to Do It:

1. Wrap a belt or strap around the ankle and thigh of your bent right leg, holding the ends with your right hand. Place the sole of your right foot at the top of your left inner thigh, bringing the foot as high up the leg as possible. With your left hand, hold on to a chair or wall. Press your right knee back, trying to bring it in line with your right hip.

2. Gaze at a spot on the floor, but keep your eyes soft. Breathe gently.

3. If you feel steady in this position, try lifting your left hand a few inches off the chair. Hold the position for 3 or 4 breaths. Don't worry if you sway or wobble. Simply lean on the chair or wall to regain your balance before trying again.

4. Bring your right foot down slowly, letting the belt slip off your leg (control the motion). Stand steady with both feet firmly grounded.

5. Repeat on the other side.

EAGLE POSE *(GARUDASANA)*

What It Does: Eagle Pose is a standing meditation that promotes mindfulness and calm. Practicing it will stretch the shoulder blades, arms, and hands; strengthen the legs; and improve balance and stamina. Practice the arm and leg sequences separately until you can maintain control, alignment, and balance. Stand near a chair or wall in case you need a little support.

How to Do It:

1. Practice Eagle arms first. Stand straight with arms extended out to the sides in a T position. Cross your left arm under your right and join your palms together.

Feel the stretch across your shoulders and upper back. Breathe softly and hold.

2. Repeat, this time crossing right arm under the left.

3. Now Practice Eagle legs. Stand straight near a chair or wall in case you need a little support. Bend your knees, then cross your right leg over your left and hook your right ankle around the back of your left ankle. If you have difficulty hooking the right ankle behind the left ankle, simply lower your right foot so the tops of the toes rest on the floor. Breathe softly and balance for a few seconds. Then release to standing straight.

4. Repeat, this time crossing the left leg over the right.

5. When you feel you can maintain control, combine the arm and leg sequences together. Stand straight, arms outstretched in T position. Cross your left arm under your right, joining palms together. Bend your knees, then cross and wrap your right leg over your left and hook your right ankle around the back of your left ankle. If you have difficulty with this second cross, simply lower your right foot so the tops of the toes rest on the floor. Breathe and balance!

6. Repeat, reversing the cross of the arms and legs.

HALF LORD OF THE FISHES POSE
(ARDHA MATSYENDRASANA)

What It Does: Half Lord of the Fishes Pose relieves emotional, mental, and physical tension and anxiety.

How to Do It:

1. Kneel, then rest your buttocks on the backs of your heels. Place your left hand on the floor and gently shift your weight down to the left until your sit bones rest on the mat to the left of your feet. Cross your right leg over your left knee, so that the right foot is flat on the floor alongside the left knee and the left foot is resting against the back of the right thigh. Then place the fingertips of your right hand on the floor, behind your right buttock.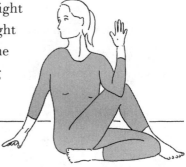

2. Exhale, twisting your torso, and place your left arm and elbow against the outer right thigh. Bend your left arm, pressing it against the right lower thigh. The fingertips reach toward the ceiling. Gaze over your right shoulder.

3. Inhale and lengthen the spine up. Exhale and deepen the twist to the right. Focus on your breathing. Hold the pose for several breaths.

4. Release and repeat on the other side.

CROCODILE TWIST POSE
(JATHARA PARIVARTANASANA VARIATION)

What It Does: Crocodile Twist relieves emotional, mental, and physical tension and anxiety. The pose takes its name from the arm movements reminiscent of the opening and closing of a crocodile's jaws.

How to Do It:

1. Begin by lying on your left side, with your right knee bent and your right foot resting on your left knee. Both arms are extended to the left; palms are together.

2. Inhale, raising the right arm and reaching and opening to the right, until the

arm rests on the mat (opening the crocodile's jaws). Palms face up to the ceiling. Turn your head and look over your right shoulder.

3. Exhale and press the shoulder blades into the mat. In this position, your right knee will have come slightly off the mat.

4. Inhale and stretch your arms further in the T position. Exhale and place your left hand on your right knee, gently pressing it to the floor, deepening the twist to the right. Focus on your breathing. With each of the next 3 inhalations, increase the stretch of the arms, and with each exhalation deepen the twist to the right.

5. Come out of the pose by bringing the right arm back to the beginning position, joining the left arm, with palms together (closing the crocodile's jaws). Lie on your left side.

6. Repeat on the opposite side.

MODIFIED HEAD-TO-KNEE POSE
(MODIFIED JANU SIRSASANA)

What It Does: Modified Head-to-Knee Pose is calming and relaxing, and it counteracts anxiety and insomnia. This pose increases the flexibility and strength of the spine, hips, and legs and tones the abdomen and abdominal organs. As you grow more flexible, you can dispense with the belt and the blanket.

How to Do It:

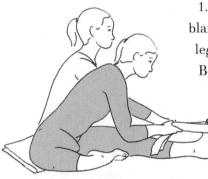

1. Sit on the floor, with a folded blanket under your hips and your legs stretched out in front of you. Bend your right leg and rest the sole of your right foot against your left thigh. Wrap a belt or strap around the ball of your left foot and fully extend your arms.

2. Inhale and lengthen your torso, pulling up from the waist. Press your shoulder blades down.

3. Exhale and fold forward, leading with the sternum and rotating to the left in order to center your torso over your straight left leg. Allow your pelvis to rotate forward. Spine stays straight. Don't curve the upper back as you reach forward. If you feel pain or discomfort in your back or leg, bend your left leg as much as necessary to alleviate it. Never force yourself.

4. Inhale and elongate your spine, lengthening your torso forward. Exhale and stretch to your edge, the point beyond which you would feel discomfort. Work up to holding for 2 or 3 breaths.

5. Inhale and come up slowly. Repeat on the other side.

YOGA ROCK AND ROLL

What It Does: Yoga Rock and Roll tones the nervous system and helps eliminate stress and tensions that may interfere with sleep. Practice this pose on a rug or a padded mat.

How to Do It:

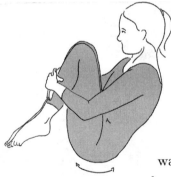

1. Sit up straight with knees bent and feet flat on the floor. Shift your weight slightly back onto your sit bones, bring your knees to your chest, and give yourself a hug. Slightly round your back.

2. Inhale, then exhale and rock backward on rounded spine, from buttocks to shoulders. Inhale and rock forward, back up

to sitting. Repeat the rock and roll 6 times, inhaling as you rock up and exhaling as you rock back.

3. Now rest on your back. Observe the sensations that follow. Does your back feel warm and relaxed?

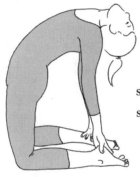

CAMEL POSE *(USTRASANA)*

What It Does: Camel Pose tones the nervous system and helps eliminate stress and tensions that may interfere with sleep. It is an excellent stretch for the front of the thighs and the back.

How to Do It:

1. Kneel on a mat, with knees about 6 inches apart. Place your hands on your lower back with fingers pointing down. To protect your lower back, tighten your buttocks and tuck your pelvis under. Drop your head back comfortably.

2. Inhale and lean back, arching your spine and squeezing your shoulder blades together. If you don't feel ready to continue, stop at this point.

3. Release your right hand from your lower back and grasp your right heel, then release your left hand and grasp your left heel. As you grow more practiced, release both hands and grasp the heels at the same time.

4. Exhale and tighten your buttocks, pressing your pelvis forward. Inhale and lift your chest toward the ceiling. Hold for 2 breaths.

5. To come out of the pose, release your hands from your heels. Leading with your pelvis, use your thigh muscles to slowly return to kneeling erect.

6. Sit on your heels and relax.

Index

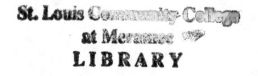

About the Author

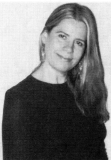

ELAINE GAVALAS received her master's degree from Columbia University, New York. She's an exercise physiologist, health expert, and weight management specialist. Elaine works with groups and with individuals of all sizes, shapes, and ages to help them reach and maintain their ideal weight, wellness, and fitness goals. She utilizes yoga and fitness techniques that integrate the body, mind, and spirit.

Elaine's Yoga Minibook series includes *The Yoga Minibook for Weight Loss, The Yoga Minibook for Stress Relief, The Yoga Mini-book for Longevity,* and *The Yoga Minibook for Energy and Strength.* Gavalas is also the author of numerous yoga, fitness, and diet articles and books, including *Secrets of Fat-Free Greek Cooking* (Penguin Putnam Avery, 1998).

If you or your company would like to contact Elaine or want more information about her books, videotapes, or group and individual services, visit her website at www.yogaminibooks.com or e-mail her at AskElaineG@ aol.com.

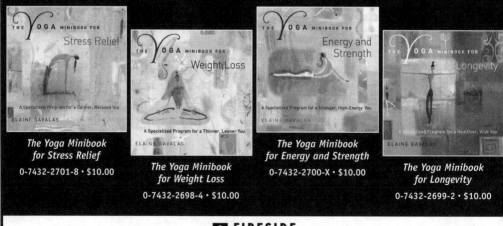